1676

Low Birth Weight:
A Medical, Psychological,
and Social Study

Low Birth Weight: A Medical, Psychological, and Social Study

Edited by

Raymond Illsley
Director of the Medical Research Council
Medical Sociology Unit, Aberdeen

and

Ross G. Mitchell
Professor of Child Health, University of Dundee

A Wiley Medical Publication

JOHN WILEY AND SONS
Chichester · New York · Brisbane · Toronto · Singapore

Library of Congress Cataloging in Publication Data:
Main entry under title:

Low birth weight.

  (A Wiley medical publication)
  Includes index.
  1. Birth weight, Low—Scotland—Aberdeen (Grampian)—
Longitudinal studies. 2. Child development—Scotland—
Aberdeen (Grampian)—Longitudinal studies. I. Illsley,
Raymond. II. Mitchell, Ross G. III. Series. [DNLM:
1; Infant, Low birth weight. WS 420 L912]
RJ281.L68 1984   618.92'01   83-16963

ISBN 0 471 90355 8

British Library Cataloguing in Publication Data:

Low birth weight—(A Wiley medical publication)
  1. Infants (Premature)   2. Birth weight
  I. Illsley, R.   II. Mitchell, Ross G.
  618.92'011   RJ250

ISBN 0 471 90355 8

Set by MHL Typesetting Limited, Coventry
and printed by St Edmundsbury Press, Bury St Edmunds, Suffolk

Acknowledgements

During the fifteen years between 1966 and 1981 a great many people and organizations played a part in this research study by contributing advice, facilities or direct help. To all of them we express our warmest thanks: the complete list is too long to record here but those concerned in the follow-up study are referred to in Chapter 6. We are particularly grateful to those colleagues who participated in the work at various stages and whose names do not appear in the list of principal contributors to this book. They are Mr William Bytheway, Prof. K.J. Dennis, Dr Elizabeth Duthie, Miss Linda Feldman, Mrs Ruth Graham, Mrs Shirley Hart, Mrs Lesley Inglis, Mrs Margo Kreckel, Dr K. Mackay, Mrs Helen Matthews, Mrs Muriel Milne, Mr Ben Sauvé and Dr Fiona Wilson.

We are also pleased to acknowledge help from the nursing staff of Aberdeen Maternity Hospital and to express our thanks to Professor Ian MacGillivray and Professor A.G.M. Campbell of the University of Aberdeen, both of whom gave much personal and departmental support.

The study was made possible by generous financial support from Action for the Crippled Child, the Medical Research Council, and the Scottish Home and Health Department.

Finally we thank our secretaries, Miss Anne Forbes, Mrs Jeanette Thorn and Mrs Betty Forsyth, for their invaluable help in the preparation of this book.

RAYMOND ILLSLEY
ROSS MITCHELL

List of Contributors

ROY CARR-HILL, B.A., Dip.Soc.Admin., M.Crim., D.Phil., Social Statistician, Medical Research Council Medical Sociology Unit, Aberdeen.

Responsible for the derivation of sociological indices and the final analysis of the relationship between the medical, social, and psychological data.

JOHN CATER, M.D., F.R.C.P.Ed., D.C.H., Senior Lecturer in Child Health, University of Dundee: formerly Research Fellow, Department of Child Health, University of Aberdeen.

Responsible for the medical and neurological study of the infants.

CYNTHIA FRASER, M.A., Dip.Ed., Psychologist, Medical Research Council Medical Sociology Unit, Aberdeen.

Responsible for the psychological testing and analysis of results at the age of 10 years.

MARGARET GILL, M.B., Ch.B., Research Medical Officer, Department of Child Health, University of Dundee.

Responsible for the medical examinations at the age of 10 years.

ANGELA HEWITT, M.A., Secretary and Administrative Officer, Medical Research Council Medical Sociology Unit, Aberdeen.

Responsible for tracing the families and making arrangements for the follow-up study.

RAYMOND ILLSLEY, C.B.E., B.A., Ph.D., Director of the Medical Research Council Medical Sociology Unit, Aberdeen.

Responsible for the sociological part of the study.

ROSS MITCHELL, M.D., F.R.C.P.Ed., D.C.H., Professor of Child Health, University of Dundee: formerly Professor of Child Health, University of Aberdeen.

Responsible for initiating the low birth weight study.

MARION RUSSELL, B.Sc., Research Officer, Medical Research Council Medical Sociology Unit, Aberdeen.

Responsible to Professor Illsley for the organization, preparation, and basic analysis of the sociological data.

MIKE SAMPHIER, B.Sc. (Econ.), Sociologist, Medical Research Council Medical Sociology Unit, Aberdeen.

Responsible for the design of coding frames and the computerization of data.
BARBARA THOMPSON, B.A., Dip.Soc.Studies, Ph.D., Social Scientist, Medical Research Council Medical Sociology Unit, Aberdeen.

Responsible for the co-ordination of both the follow-up study and the preparation of the final report.

Contents

Foreword

by SIR DUGALD BAIRD,
Emeritus Professor of Obstetrics and
Gynaecology in the University of Aberdeen

Great progress has been made in the last 50 years in making childbirth safer for mother and baby. In the United Kingdom, maternal mortality fell rapidly in the 1930s, basically as a result of the successful treatment of puerperal sepsis. Stillbirths were first notifiable in 1928 but little fall in the perinatal mortality rate (PMR) occurred till the Second World War with improvement in maternal diets as a result of food rationing. In the years 1948–60, the first 12 years of the National Health Service, the fall in the PMR from better obstetric care was largely offset by a rise in the death rates from low birth weight (LBW) and malformations of the central nervous system, resulting from the poor reproductive efficiency of mothers born during the economic depression of the late 1920s and early 1930s. The steady fall in the PMR since the early 1960s has resulted from improvement in the obstetric and paediatric services and in the reproductive efficiency of young mothers born during and after the war.

Since 1976 the fall in the rate has been more rapid in all social classes but the class differences still remain. In Scotland as late as 1981, in single births and excluding all deaths from congenital malformations, 66% of all perinatal deaths were in LBW babies—i.e. those weighing 2500 g or less at birth—and in over 60% of these no clinical 'cause' was found. The large contribution made to the PMR by these LBW infants, who comprise only about 7% of births, and the increased survival rate in LBW babies of all weights has led to many studies of their subsequent health and development.

In this book the authors attempt to unravel the relationship between birth weight, its antecedents and external influences during childhood on physical, intellectual and emotional development of all LBW babies in a total, geographically defined population. For this purpose a carefully matched control series of heavier children born as soon after each index case as possible was identified. They were matched for social class, maternal height, ordinal position, smoking habits and sex of child. The difficulties encountered in this task are described in detail.

The mothers of the LBW babies were less efficient obstetrically than those of the controls, having had more abortions, obstetric complications and maternal diseases. The socio-cultural background of the LBW mothers was much poorer in many respects. They were found to have fewer aspirations, less social contact with neighbours, a more limited range of vocabulary and less fluency of expression. These personal characteristics cannot be summarized in the form of a single indicator. Such an assessment is shown, however, to be more valuable than the husband's occupational classification, especially if the interview is conducted by a person of wide experience and the necessary personal attributes.

At the age of 10 years the LBW children were still lighter and shorter than their controls and had more neurological disorders. They showed impairment of intelligence, regardless of other factors, especially if the LBW was due to slow growth rather than short gestation. Such growth impairment in the children of tall women was more likely to suggest serious disturbance of reproductive efficiency than in those of short women. The mother who feels incompetent is more likely to create an environment less favourable to the child's development than one who is cheerful and dynamic and who may indeed be able to offset the effect of initial disadvantages.

A major conclusion of this study seems to be that the disadvantages of being of low weight at birth are largely the result of the unfavourable environment in which these children are reared, which points to the need for greater efforts to improve the home environment. How can one ensure these advantages of a stimulating environment, especially in the first five years when the brain is growing so rapidly? The authors think that allocating more resources towards research of this kind might be more productive in the long term than the over-lavish provision and equipment of hospital units.

The factors influencing reproductive efficiency of future mothers and the incidence of LBW begin to operate at a very early stage inside the mother's uterus and are more difficult to influence than the quality of the care and attention received from birth to maturity.

The greatest fall in the PMR in the last 20 years has occurred in fifth and later births to women in social classes IV and V. The fact that very few women in these classes now have more than two children should make it easier for such mothers today to give their children 'a good start in life'. Possibly these mothers will be more cheerful and dynamic than their predecessors. Such changes in reproductive habits could not have occurred at a better time when we seem to be facing many years of high unemployment.

The investigations described in this book required a favourable setting, easy access to a total population and team work involving several disciplines. These requirements have been met, which makes this study from Aberdeen most valuable and instructive, especially to those working in this field.

List of Tables

List of Figures

Note

Throughout this book, reference is made to the Registrar-General's classification of the population by Social Class.

In the United Kingdom, the Registrar-General classifies Social Class according to father's occupation into:

I   Professional
II   Intermediate
III   Skilled
IV   Partially skilled
V   Unskilled.

For present purposes, Social Class III is subdivided into:

IIIa   Non-manual
IIIb   Journeyman occupations (i.e. requiring a time-served apprenticeship)
IIIc   Remainder of skilled manual occupations.

In some places, IIIb and IIIc have been combined as IIIb.

Chapter 1

Introduction to the Aberdeen Low Birth Weight Study

R. ILLSLEY AND R.G. MITCHELL

There have been many changes during the last half century in the reproductive habits of populations, the technology and management of childbirth, and the care of newborn infants. Throughout this period, birth weight has been, as it continues to be, a central focus of professional and social interest. The essential source of concern lies in the implications of birth weight, and particularly of low birth weight (LBW), for the survival of infants and for the later physical and mental health and development of children.

The nature of the problem has changed over the years. Initially, in the more affluent societies the rate of LBW fell and this contributed substantially to a fall in the numbers of stillbirths and early infant deaths. Since the 1950s, however, the rate of LBW has remained fairly constant in Britain and in many other developed countries. The reasons are still obscure, for it might have been expected that the rate would fall under the joint influence of an increased coverage of antenatal care and an improvement in living standards. Moreover, the greatest falls in perinatal death rates have occurred amongst babies within the normal range of birth weight, so that LBW babies with their lower and less improved survival rates have constituted an ever-increasing proportion of perinatal deaths. In Scotland in 1981, the 6 per cent of LBW babies accounted for 67 per cent of perinatal deaths. Numerically, perinatal death comes more and more to mean the death of LBW babies.

At the same time one significant change has been the increased survival rate amongst babies of very low birth weight (VLBW) and this has given further grounds for anxiety about the relationship between birth weight and later impairment of neurodevelopmental functioning. Previous studies have attempted to address the question: 'Do LBW babies perform less well in later life than heavier babies, either in physical development and health or in intellectual abilities?' The longitudinal study which is the subject of this book was designed to throw light on that same question and is therefore the successor to a number of investigations, the results of which are summarized in Chapter 2. Some of the earliest studies were concerned solely with weight at birth. Later thought emphasized the possibility that weight alone might be a misleading criterion and that account should be taken of the stage of gestation at which babies were delivered. Thus total groups of LBW babies were subdivided in various ways to indicate whether babies were light (or very light) for the stage of gestation, were at an appropriate weight for gestational age at delivery (for comparison with babies delivered at term and within the normal range of birth weight) or were born very early. These considerations are also addressed in the present study.

One of the most difficult problems in the design and interpretation of studies of this kind is to make due allowance for factors other than birth weight (or factors interacting with weight) known to influence the subsequent development of children. To minimize that interpretative problem, our study compares LBW children with a sample of children who were heavier at birth and with whom they were matched on five variables (maternal height, ordinal position, parental social class, mother's smoking habits, and sex of child) known to affect the weight, growth, and social and intellectual development of children. The procedures by which 149 matched pairs of LBW and control children were chosen, the implications of that procedure and its limitations are discussed in Chapter 3.

Information on the characteristics of the parents and the socio-cultural environment of the family into which the child was born was obtained by interview with the mother three weeks after the birth. Matching procedures using such indirect indicators of the environment as social class and family size do not eliminate socio-cultural differences. The information collected at interview after the birth was needed to examine the possibility that differences in physical and intellectual development might be due to residual socio-cultural influences on the child. Chapter 4 describes the procedure by which such potential influences were identified and combined in a range of composite indices. It was not feasible to collect further detailed information on the environment and social experience of the children at subsequent stages—a gap in our knowledge which adds to problems of interpretation.

Both the LBW and the control children were intensively studied by a paediatrician in the period immediately after birth: the children were re-examined by the same doctor at the age of 10 months. The purpose was to identify congenital and neonatal problems likely to have a significant effect on later development and also to examine the sub-categories of weight and gestational age to see whether at these ages their developmental profiles differed significantly. The scope of these investigations and a summary of results are presented in Chapter 5, and more fully by Cater (1978).

The study was based on all LBW children born in the Aberdeen area over a specified period, together with their matched controls. It was decided to trace and re-examine these children at the age of 10 years—an age at which comprehensive and reliable measures could be applied and by which differences in development would have emerged. To avoid selective bias in the results it was important to trace as many children as possible. We describe in Chapter 6 the complex process by which LBW and control samples were traced and through which it became possible to interview 282 out of the original sample of 298 children.

Re-examination at 10 years involved two major components: a medical developmental examination conducted mainly by a part-time medical practitioner in collaboration with the paediatrician who had examined the children at birth and at 10 months and a psychological examination conducted by a full-time research psychologist. Neither the medical practitioner nor the psychologist was informed about the birth weight status of the children before they carried out their examinations. The procedure and the results of these examinations are presented in Chapters 7 and 8.

The final stage, presented in Chapter 9, brings together the results of these medical, sociological, and psychological investigations conducted at birth, in the neonatal period, at 10 months and at 10 years. It is thus possible to relate birth weight and factors associated with it to medical and psychological outcomes and to make allowance for the possibly complicating effect of some of the differences in the socio-cultural environment of the children.

A major problem of longitudinal study is that in the interval between commencement and conclusion of fieldwork, knowledge emerges in the scientific world which, had it been known earlier, should have been incorporated in the design and in the first stage of data collection. The investigators themselves are also likely to become a little wiser over the intervening years. This sometimes means that precise and highly discriminating end-results have to be compared with original data of lesser refinement within a design which could clearly, with hindsight, have been bettered. We believe that there are limitations to the matched control design and we refer to this in later discussion. More important, however, was the impracticability of collecting useful data between birth and the age of 10 years on the actual social environment and experience of the children and their families. Nevertheless, we would argue that these omissions do not invalidate our findings of differences or lack of differences between the LBW and control groups or the sub-categories of the LBW population and that these are of considerable interest in their own right.

Chapter 2

The Developing Concept of Low Birth Weight and the Present State of Knowledge

R. ILLSLEY AND R.G. MITCHELL

THE BACKGROUND

Reports from many countries over the last 30 years have confirmed beyond doubt the fact that low birth weight (LBW) infants who survive into childhood are more likely than heavier infants to suffer from impaired functioning. Relationships have been reliably established between LBW and congenital malformations, neurological abnormalities, mental retardation, low intellectual and educational achievement, childhood illness, and poor physical development. However, the mere demonstration of a relationship between a category of births and a variety of abnormalities in childhood says little about the causative processes involved. Although some causal connections have been demonstrated which link intra-uterine and perinatal conditions to particular outcomes, many, and perhaps the most far-reaching, questions remain unanswered. Some of these questions relate to the definition and significance of birth weight itself. LBW is conventionally defined as 2500g or less. Within this general category variations in weight itself are wide, from babies of 1500g and less to babies of 2251–2500g. The combined stillbirth and neonatal death rates of these two extreme groups in Scotland in 1978 were 776 and 29 per 1000 births (Scottish Home and Health Department, 1979). How far do the different risks of mortality imply different risks of handicap in the surviving child? The question becomes more important as the application of skilled obstetric and paediatric care leads to the survival of more babies of very low birth weight (VLBW).

Responding to an article about the improved survival rate of very small babies a correspondent in the *British Medical Journal* (Brown, 1977) raised the question in a stark form by asking how far this was a triumph of neonatal paediatrics or a 'social and family disaster' passed on by medicine to be handled by others. VLBW babies are also likely to be born prematurely and the further question arises as to whether deleterious consequences result from early delivery or from low weight at birth. Amalgamation of the two questions has led to the use of rather more sophisticated classifications concerning the 'appropriateness' of the birth weight for the duration of gestation with the assumed corollary that consequences may differ for those who are light-for-dates and appropriate-for-dates or may vary continuously across contours defined by weight and gestation (Goldstein and Peckham, 1976). The fundamental point is that different combinations of weight and gestation may reflect intra-uterine and perinatal processes and experiences, each of which may have specific implications for fetal development, for neonatal morbidity and for childhood functioning. The need to specify these parameters precisely, to identify the physiological, neurological, and biochemical processes with which they are associated, and to relate them to equally precise and specific measures of outcome has posed stringent requirements upon research design which have rarely been met.

A further broad set of questions centres around the relationship between prenatal, intranatal, and postnatal experiences. LBW does not occur randomly within and across populations. Its epidemiology suggests a disproportionate incidence in less affluent regions, in lower socio-economic groups, in first and high order births, in very young and in elderly women, and in those of short stature and of low educational achievement. These are characteristics associated with poverty and with the culture of lower class populations in industrialized societies. Many of the presumed abnormal characteristics of LBW children are also common characteristics of children brought up in relatively deprived conditions, irrespective of their birth weight. This raises the further, and most difficult, question of how far birth weight as such has any intrinsic effect on childhood development and functioning. One extreme of this argument would suggest that low weight at birth and poor development in childhood are each separate manifestations of relative deprivation which are associated because the parents, whose past experiences of deprivation have led to the birth of an LBW child, bring up that child in a lifestyle which reflects their own deprivation. LBW children, on this hypothesis, are more likely than heavier babies to have sub-optimal diets, to be subjected to the risks of infection and accidents, to have inadequate medical care, to lack intellectual stimulation and a drive towards achievement, and to receive low standards of formal and informal education. A less extreme, interactionist, variant of this argument would suggest that an unfavourable environment reinforces any intrinsic birth weight effect and equally that a favourable environment may compensate fully or partially for a birth weight disadvantage. On this hypothesis the outcome for LBW children in the upper social groups should not differ greatly from that of their heavier peers.

Testing for the applicability of these alternative hypotheses, as with the previous and related set of issues, requires various bodies of carefully recorded observation over a long period of time.

1. The first body of data is required to answer the question: How do the parents of LBW children differ from each other and from the parents of heavier children in characteristics likely to affect birth weight and gestation and subsequently to affect the physical, intellectual, and social development of their children? This may be briefly described as the social epidemiology of LBW.
2. The second body of data relates to the events of pregnancy, labour and delivery. Such data should be sufficient to categorize the population in terms of birth weight, gestation, major complications of pregnancy, and significant differences in the modes of delivery.
3. The third set of data relates to the condition of the child at birth and in the early neonatal period and is required to differentiate between children at birth as distinct from the events of pregnancy and to identify early signs of abnormality or of postnatal experience likely to have implications for future development.
4. The fourth body of data relates to the social and medical experience of the child from the neonatal period through to the point(s) at which levels of functioning are assessed and needs to be focused upon experiences which are, by themselves or in combination with other events and conditions, likely to affect the development of health status and of intellectual and social functioning.
5. The final body of data consists of the battery of descriptions, measurements and assessments which constitute outcome. Ideally outcome should be assessed at several points in childhood, partly to differentiate between transitory and permanent abilities and disabilities and partly to coincide with major anticipated stages in social experience, e.g. before and after school entry.

Given these exacting requirements it is not surprising that so many investigators have attempted short cuts. The following are typical of such strategies:

1. The retrospective documentation of Stages 1, 2 or 3 above, i.e. the epidemiology of LBW and/or of the circumstances of the pregnancy, delivery, and neonatal periods, using either maternal recall or more frequently case records not specifically compiled for research purposes.

2. The omission of any direct information under Stage 4, i.e. postnatal experience, data being collected retrospectively by interview or questionnaire at the point of final outcome.
3. The reliance on indirect data at Stage 5, e.g. use of classifications of height, weight or IQ obtained for all schoolchildren as part of the routine of the school system.
4. The use of small samples of clinical case material rather than systematic sampling of total populations, or the accumulation of samples over long periods of time with children being assessed at very different ages.

As a result of these economizing strategies it is often possible to relate two or three of the necessary bodies of data but only a few studies contain the comprehensive material necessary for a complete analysis. In the following review, disproportionate attention has therefore been paid to a few studies, viz, the Baltimore studies associated with Knobloch and Pasamanick (Knobloch *et al.*, 1956); the Newcastle study carried out by Neligan and his colleagues (1976); the follow-up of the 1946 Maternity Survey of Great Britain carried out by J.W.B. Douglas (Douglas and Gear, 1976); and the British Perinatal Mortality Study and its follow-up carried out by Butler and his colleagues (Davie *et al.*, 1972). The findings in this field of study have been frequently and fully reviewed (e.g. by Birch and Gussow, 1970) and we do not therefore consider it necessary to preface this work with another comprehensive review. Instead we shall focus, under each of the five stages of research, upon well-established findings and use them for two purposes, to identify gaps in knowledge and to discuss problems of interpretation which arise in the relationship between stages.

SOCIAL EPIDEMIOLOGY OF LOW BIRTH WEIGHT

Social class

Many social variables can be shown to be positively correlated with birth weight. The problem arises in the interpretation of their aetiological significance. In a study of indicator variables across 21 countries, Boldman and Reed (1977) produced sizeable correlations between LBW and urban residence, per capita income, per capita energy consumption, population per physician, and newspaper circulation and radio and TV ownership per 1000 population. However, these indicators were themselves strongly intercorrelated and the investigators were able to show that 70 per cent of the observed variation could be attributed to differences in per capita income, the further items each adding little to the explanation. Similarly, within particular countries, correlations can be demonstrated with a range of maternal background characteristics such as area of residence, housing conditions, educational level, marital status, unemployment, the occupations of the mother, her husband, and her father, and social and geographical mobility, as well as with more directly health-related factors such as week of first attendance at the antenatal clinic. Some of these correlations are clearly spurious in that there are no logical reasons for linking the indicator to either fetal growth or premature delivery. Most of the individual correlations are reduced to insignificance when they are controlled against the most general indicator of social status, i.e. the classification of either maternal or paternal occupation into socio-economic groups. Regrettably, the only plausible conclusion which can be drawn from the great volume of studies employing such social indicators is both speculative and highly general in nature. The best social predictors of LBW in a population are those which most efficiently summarize the net results of the exposure of the mother over many years of childhood and early adult life to living conditions associated with the material conditions and life style of poverty. Social class is an intellectual and social construct; it has no material form and cannot directly affect the development of the fetus in its uterine environment or cause its premature expulsion. Yet its relationship with so many aspects of child and adult illness and death (Black, 1980; Birch and Gussow, 1970) shows that it nevertheless has biological significance. Summarizing their comprehensive review of the health, nutrition, and school achievement of disadvantaged children, Birch and Gussow (1970) emphasize social position as a factor which continuously and cumulatively influences the exposure of the individual to other and more direct causes of health and ill-health:

> ... the environments in which disadvantaged children develop from conception on are far less supportive to growth and health than are those of children who are not disadvantaged, and this relative environmental impoverishment is exaggerated when the disadvantaged child is non-white.. The differences are profound and prolonged. Mothers of such children tend to be less well fed, less well grown, and less well cared for before they reach childbearing age. When they reach it, they begin to bear children younger, more rapidly, and more often, and they continue to bear them to an older age. When such a mother is pregnant both her nutrition and her health will tend to be poorer than that of a woman who is better off, but she will be far less likely to get prenatal care and far more likely to be delivered under substandard conditions.
>
> Children of such mothers are smaller at birth, die more readily, and are generally in poorer condition in infancy than are children born to the more affluent. If they survive the first month of life their mortality thereafter is excessively high and their illnesses more frequent, more persistent, and more severe. Their early nutrition is negatively influenced by their mother's health, her age, her income level, her education, her habits and attitudes, so that among such children in the preschool years frank malnutrition, as well as subclinical manifestations of depressed nutritional status (reflected in anaemia and poor growth), are markedly more prevalent. During the school years they eat irregularly, their health care continues to be almost totally inadequate, their housing is substandard, their family income is low, subsistence on public assistance is high, and family disorganization common-place.

Social class (like 'environment') thus emerges as an indicator of other and more direct influences whose significance varies with the context in which it is employed. In relation to birth weight its significance lies in its ability, in one measurement, to encapsulate all those past experiences in the life of a mother which have affected her biological functioning as a reproductive agent. If no relationship exists in a given society between social class and birth weight it either means that, in that society, women of different social classes do not have differential exposure to health-related influences (there are suggestions, for example, that this may now be the case in Sweden) or, more probably, that the measure of social class employed does not efficiently encapsulate the woman's relevant past experience (this may be the reason why occupational position and birth weight do not appear to be correlated in present day Cuba (WHO, 1978)).

If, on the other hand, we consider the relationship between social class and the level of a child's educational achievement, social class has a quite different significance. Social class in these circumstances relates most directly to the cultural and intellectual exposure of the child through the type of stimulation provided by parents and peers and through the quality of educational provision. There may, of course, be some biological component in the relationship, in so far as the child's health may itself have an impact on intellectual achievement, but in most circumstances this is likely to be secondary to the direct impact of the cultural environment.

This interpretation of social class as a multiple indicator, whose relevance varies with the context of its use, has important implications for the interpretation of the relationship between birth weight and the child's intellectual, educational, and social functioning. In dealing with maternal social class and birth weight the most relevant dimension of social class is biological—its ability to summarize the effect of maternal social experience from birth to maturity upon the woman's reproductive efficiency. This in itself, however, may only be a weak indicator of the child's postnatal environment, for it relies upon the assumption that parents in each social class will provide an environmental upbringing for their child which has a strong rank correlation with the environment which produced them a generation earlier. Although such a correlation does exist, inter-generational social mobility is substantial. Parents in Social Class V may therefore provide a Class III environment for their children and vice versa (Illsley, 1980). This suggests very strongly that assessment of the child's background must be based upon observation of that specific background and that the parent's social class cannot be reliably used as a proxy indicator.

Maternal height

From the early 1950s onwards, Baird and his colleagues in Aberdeen began to show that the following three relationships existed:

1. A relationship between social class and height—women in lower social classes being shorter in stature than those in upper social classes.

2. A relationship between women's height and the birth weight of their children—shorter women producing smaller babies.
3. A relationship between social class and birth weight—women from lower social classes producing smaller babies.

These findings have been subsequently confirmed for national populations (Butler and Bonham, 1963; Butler and Alberman, 1969; Chamberlain *et al.*, 1975). Height, of course, has a strong genetic component and there are good grounds for concluding that parental height has a dominating effect on birth weight and on the height of children during their school years (Rona *et al.*, 1978). The common explanation for the class differential in stature is that environmental factors influence the ability of individuals to reach their genetic potential. Part, at least, of that environment is concerned with dietary intake during childhood. Thomson and Billewicz (1963) express the relationship as follows: 'Stature may thus be used as a statistic which reflects dietary habits during growth; and since food habits acquired during growth tend to persist, adult stature also tends to reflect nutritional status'. Social class and maternal height therefore seem to be different means of assessing during early adult life the effect of living conditions experienced in infancy and childhood and may be used as indirect indicators for a host of influences from the past which cannot be reconstructed in detail by retrospective inquiry.

These two indicators overlap but each seems to measure something not identified by the other. Thus within a given height group, substantial differences occur in the rate of LBW between social classes; and also substantial variations by height exist within social classes. The incidence of LBW in married women having a first baby rises by steps from 4.8 per cent in upper class tall women to 15.2 per cent in lower class short women (Baird, 1974; and Table 2.1.)

Table 2.1 Percentage of LBW, married primigravidae, by maternal height and social class, Aberdeen 1968–71

Social Class	Tall 163 cm and over	% LBW Medium 155–162 cm	Small less than 155 cm
I–III a	4.8	4.0	13.8
III b	4.8	5.7	11.1
IV and V	7.0	9.7	15.2

If other potentially influencing factors are added so that the total index of maternal background becomes more fully reflective of the individual's history, greater discrimination is likely to occur. Baird (1974) used an assessment of physique and health recorded at the first antenatal visit and this produced sharp differentiation in LBW rates with height groups. In an analysis of perinatal mortality Illsley (1966) showed that the addition of data about region of residence in Britain led to additional discrimination within social class and height groups.

In using data on maternal physique to explain variations in children's heights, it should be remembered that, as with social class, the factors which determined maternal physique apply only partially to their children. Davie *et al.* (1972) show that, even having allowed for maternal social class and height, factors specific to the child's history (particularly birth order and the number of younger siblings) had quite a substantial additional influence. This again stresses the need to assess the child's environment separately from long-term maternal characteristics.

Parity and maternal age

In what has now become a classic study, Morris and Heady (1955) showed the complex relationship between stillbirths and neonatal and post-neonatal mortality and maternal age and parity. This pointed very strongly to a combination of biological and social factors in the risks of death. More recently, related data on LBW have emerged (Butler and Bonham, 1963; Donnelly *et al.*, 1964; Birch and Gussow, 1970). The results show a remarkably stable pattern. For each parity LBW rates tend to be high in teenage mothers, reach a low point in the late twenties, and rise after 35 years of age—the peaks and troughs varying slightly for each parity but always showing a U-shaped curve. At each age there is a constant pattern of high rates for first parity births, low rates for second and third parity births, with rates rising in the fourth and subsequent parities. Within these categories the usual social class gradient applies, but there is a clear tendency for the rise with age to occur earlier in the lower social groups.

The statistical facts, now widely reported, are not in dispute, but there is much uncertainty about their meaning. Again the basic question concerns the relative contributions of biological and social factors. On the biological hypothesis, the curve with age represents physiological immaturity in the teens and maturity in the twenties followed by physiological ageing in the thirties. The curve with parity represents, on the same hypothesis, a physiological running-in problem, followed by an absence of complications and then by a mixture of ageing and an overburdening of the reproductive system. The social hypothesis, on the other hand, emphasizes the differing specific socio-biological composition of each combination of age and parity, pointing to the tendency for women who bear children very early to be drawn from the most disadvantaged groups (even within a single social class) and to the progressive social selectivity of higher parity groups and higher age groups. This interpretation gains support from a recent analysis of the obstetric histories of a cohort of 13 322 women whose pregnancies have all resulted in a live-born baby of certain gestation. In this admittedly selected group there is a distinct tendency for birth weights to increase slightly with each further pregnancy when account has been taken of the related factors—maternal age, parity, height, social class, sex of baby, and birth interval (Carr-Hill and Samphier, personal communication). This result stems from the analysis of successive pregnancies to the same women, as opposed to the cross-sectional analysis of births at varying ages and parities to different women—a method which ignores the changing composition of age and parity groups.

The implications of these two interpretations for the relationship between maternal characteristics, birth weight and later child functioning are important. On the biological hypothesis, age/parity differentials in LBW are largely a function of the intra-uterine environment; on the social hypothesis they have direct implications for the family environment in which the child will be reared and therefore properly belong to that set of factors which directly influence the postnatal environment.

Implications of the social epidemiology of LBW for the later functioning of children

The time-scale of research work on LBW and its effects has militated against the inclusion of more than a few conventional variables reflecting the pre-pregnancy characteristics of the mother (and almost no data are available on fathers). The two major studies which examine the whole range of pre-pregnancy, pregnancy, perinatal, and postnatal influences show the relationship of child functioning to social class (based on the father's occupation), maternal height, age, parity, and smoking.

The indicators of functioning examined by Davie, Butler, and Goldstein (1972) include reading attainment, social or behavioural adjustment at school as assessed by teachers, and the child's height. The main factors, in descending order, related to child's height (with separate allowance for the effect of other factors) were: birth order, maternal height, birth weight, social class, number of younger siblings, smoking during pregnancy, and age of the mother. The biological factors of maternal height and birth weight had a clear and substantial influence. So also did birth order, height decreasing with birth order and with the number of younger siblings, and the authors attribute this relationship to the competition for resources in larger families. Social class had a lesser, though still significant and recognizable effect. For reading attainment, however, social class had the major effect, followed closely by birth order and the number of younger siblings, the birth weight effect being small. For social adjustment the major factors were social class, birth order, smoking, length of gestation, and number of younger siblings; maternal age, birth weight, and maternal height made relatively small additional contributions. The authors, well aware of the effect of smoking on birth weight itself, were puzzled about its effect on social adjustment of the child; their findings on gestational age will be considered in more detail later. Perhaps the most revealing point for our purposes is that the predominantly postnatal influences—birth order, number of younger siblings, and social class—have a clear and substantial impact upon biological, intellectual, and social outcomes, whereas the biological factors—maternal height and birth weight—only contribute substantially to the child's height.

Neligan and his co-workers (1976) looked at a range of physical, neurological, intellectual, and behavioural outcomes. In addition to the independent variables used by Davie, Butler, and Goldstein, they employed a measure of the mother's care of the child. Their results are complex and refer to three different populations, a random sample of all births, those who were born very prematurely, and those who were light-for-dates. In all three populations, the most important influence on a combined index of outcomes was the mother's care of the child, which clearly out-weighed social class itself and also ordinal position in the family. The mother's expectations for the child made an additional contribution. Maternal height was important as well, but less so than the family factors. The effect of birth weight was quite small. These authors sum up their results as follows: 'When the absolute and relative importance of associated factors are assessed, those we have called "biological" and "clinical" are completely overshadowed by the group of environmental factors in a representative population of children. This group we have called "family factors" because of the overwhelming importance of various attributes of the mother, and the structure of the family as a whole. Biological and clinical factors clearly affect the later performance of children in our two extreme abnormal groups to a greater extent than in our general population'. Despite the final qualification, the authors agree that even in their combined LBW group the family factors outweigh the biological and the clinical.

Two further reports deal with similar issues but, instead of concentrating on LBW, employ the whole range of birth weights. McKeown (1970), in an analysis of verbal reasoning scores for a population of 50 000 children in Birmingham, England, reports a continuous increase in scores across the range of birth weights from less than 2000 g up to 4500 g or more. He further shows that scores rise with increasing social status based on the father's occupation and that within each social group scores increase with increasing maternal age and decrease with increasing birth order. Using data on sibship pairs and on twin births, he concludes that retardation of fetal growth has little influence on measured intelligence and that the striking associations in a general population of births between measured intelligence and such variables as birth weight, duration of gestation, maternal age, and birth rank are due to postnatal influences. Illsley (1966, 1967) analysed the mean intelligence test scores at the age of 7 years for a population of 11 280 children born in Aberdeen in 1950–55. He too reports a continuous relationship of IQ with birth weight from birth weights of under $3\frac{1}{2}$ lb to 9lb. The relationship occurs within each of his four socio-economic groups (again based on the father's occupation). Taking a specific socio-economic group (skilled manual workers) he, like McKeown, found that scores increased continuously with maternal age and decreased continuously by the number of pregnancy. Within the same socio-economic group, Illsley also analysed each combined age and pregnancy group against a further index of social characteristics designed to differentiate social rankings within a socio-economic group. He showed that the ranking of age and pregnancy groups were identical for both IQ scores and for the index of social characteristics and concluded that the variations in test scores between age and number-of-pregnancy groups merely reflected hidden socio-economic differences between these groups. Analysis jointly by family size and ordinal position in the family showed that IQ scores fell continuously by family size, but that within a given family size there were no variations between different ordinal positions.

The general conclusion from these four British studies is strikingly similar, namely, that the association between birth weight and intellectual functioning reflects an association between birth weight and socio-economic status which, in turn, means that children of lower birth weights have less satisfactory postnatal environments. The study by Davie, Butler, and Goldstein (1972), however, suggests that the stature of children is jointly influenced by genetic and social factors.

BIRTH WEIGHT, LENGTH OF GESTATION AND PREGNANCY COMPLICATIONS

Birth weight and gestation

Early studies of the effect of pregnancy and perinatal factors upon childhood functioning tended to concentrate heavily upon birth weight and to ignore the possible effect of early delivery. More recently, and particularly since the publication by Thomson, Billewicz, and Hytten (1968) of centile charts relating birth weight to gestational age, the validity of using a single arbitrary cut-off point to distinguish LBW and of equating LBW with prematurity has been strongly challenged. The relatively simple and potentially misleading issue of LBW has been translated into three questions, one of which relates to the degree of LBW, one to degrees of premature delivery, and the third to degrees of growth retardation relative to the length of gestation. Research relating to these three questions is briefly reviewed below.

Goldstein and Peckham (1976) carried out a regression analysis on the data of the British National Child Development Study whose results had been more descriptively examined by Davie, Butler, and Goldstein (1972). They used three measures of mental and physical development at the age of 11 years, viz. the height of the child, the score on a reading comprehension test, and the assessed need for special schooling. Independent variables entered into the regression analysis were birth weight, length of gestation, social class, sex, number of younger and older children, and the mother's age and height. When allowance was made for the other factors they found 'a weak association for gestation and a somewhat stronger one for birth weight'. The associations differed for the different outcomes. Thus, the strongest associations for reading score were, successively, social class, the number of older children, and birth weight; the relationship with maternal height was small but significant and with length of gestation small and non-significant. For child height, the strongest associations were maternal height, birth weight, and the number of older and younger children; the association with length of gestation was again small. In relation to the need for special schooling the influence of birth weight was much greater than that of length of gestation but, because of the small number of children in need of special schooling, it was not possible to take into account the effect of associated background factors. The authors express doubts about the appropriateness of using birth-weight-for-gestation percentiles and conclude:

> For the purpose of estimating subsequent mental development, gestation length has little predictive value as compared with background variables such as social class, family size and maternal age. Similarly gestation has little value in predicting physical development when compared with birth weight, maternal height and family size.

The Goldstein analysis was concerned with relationships across the whole range of birth weights and gestation lengths and not only with LBW and early delivery. Neligan and his colleagues (1976), on the other hand, designed their study with the aim of comparing children born early (255 days or less) and children light-for-dates (below the 10th percentile) with a random sample of children. The data were analysed in two steps, the first concentrating solely upon the birth weight/gestation issue, while the second compared birth weight and gestation effects with associated background factors. The light-for-dates sample was subdivided for most purposes into very-light-for-dates children (birth weight on or below 5th centile) and rather-light-for-dates children (between 5th and 10th centiles). Leaving aside many small and specific variations, the analysis showed striking consistency in the ranking of the four groups in relation to psychometric, behavioural, neurological, and physical assessments and measurements. In all aspects of functioning the 'abnormal' groups fared significantly worse than the random controls. Similarly, the scores of the very-light-for-dates children were almost invariably 'worse' than those of the short-gestation children. The scores of the rather-light-for-dates children were never better than those of the controls, and never worse than those of the very-light-for-dates children but had a variable ranking in relation to the short-gestation group. The authors concluded that there was good evidence for supposing that the later impairment of the children was causally related to prenatal impairment of growth, in that the degree of later impairment was directly proportional to the degree of intra-uterine growth retardation in the light-for-dates sample.

While the effects of family factors were of much greater magnitude than the intra-uterine growth factor, allowance for family factors did not affect the order of ranking between the 'abnormal' groups. There is no necessary contradiction between these results and those of Goldstein quoted above, in that Neligan's data referred strictly to short gestation and intra-uterine growth retardation whereas the Goldstein analysis covered the whole range of birth weights and gestation lengths.

Questions about the degree of LBW were raised in a series of early studies before the use of birthweight-for-gestation centiles was adopted. In a review of such studies, Harper and Wiener (1965) not only confirmed the general finding that LBW children had lowered intelligence test scores but also concluded that 'three major studies using large numbers of children note progressively lower intelligence test scores with increasingly low birth weight'. Wiener's own analysis (1968) of the Baltimore data (500 'prematures' matched individually against an equivalent number of 'full-term' children matched for a variety of social and biological factors) showed the same tendency. A series of studies by Drillien (1964) reported marked lowering of scores with decreasing birth weight. Birch and Gussow (1970) concluded from their re-analysis of the Baltimore data and the studies by Drillien (1964) and McDonald (1964) that evidence to that date suggested that scores within the 'premature' group tended to decrease with decreasing birth weight. They drew attention, however, to the possibility that the rate of decrease was greater in the lowest social classes: 'Characteristically, IQ scores show a double gradient, declining as expected with social class regardless of low birth weight, and declining with birth weight within each social class group so that the most extreme differences within the premature groups occur between the IQ scores of the heaviest infants in the upper class and the lightest infants in the lower class.' These results supported Illsley's (1967) report on the Aberdeen data which suggested that birth weight had relatively little impact on IQ scores across the full range of birth weights.

The need to take account of degrees of LBW has been strengthened in recent years by the increasing survival rate of VLBW babies. While some doubt exists about the uniformity of this trend, even in centres applying the highest standards of neonatal care (Jones et al., 1979), and about the efficacy of intensive care for babies of VLBW (Steiner et al., 1980), many centres have now begun to report higher survival rates (Lancet, 1980; Stewart et al., 1981; Levene and Dubowitz, 1982). Further doubt exists about the extent to which higher survival rates in VLBW babies is accompanied by changes in the number and proportion of surviving children who have residual disabilities of varying degrees of severity. The earlier studies mentioned above sometimes excluded from consideration children with severe handicapping conditions and preferred to examine degrees of later functioning in apparently normal children. In any comprehensive study of the effects of LBW such a procedure seems questionable and potentially misleading. The more recent studies report contradictory findings on trends in the incidence of major and minor handicap in VLBW babies. A *Lancet* (1980) editorial concludes that 'it is still too early to assess the results of follow-up' in VLBW babies and points to a number of definitional and methodological problems in the design of studies and the presentation of results: following this, Kiely and Paneth (1981) made some suggestions for improving such studies. At present, the only firm conclusion must be that VLBW is accompanied by a disproportionately high rate of handicap in surviving children but that, as a result of recent improvements in intensive care, this situation may be changing.

Obstetric factors

Several studies have examined the relationship between complications of pregnancy and labour and the subsequent functioning of children in total populations of births undifferentiated by birth weight or gestation. The early Baltimore studies initiated by Pasamanick *et al.* (1956) reported associations between a range of pregnancy and perinatal complications and an equally wide range of intellectual, neurological, behavioural, and medical conditions in children. They postulated 'a continuum of reproductive casualty' whereby a range of harmful complications, sometimes (and particularly in the lower social classes) acting cumulatively, might cause death or result in one or more abnormalities in surviving children. Similar cumulative outcomes were reported by Werner *et al.* (1967) but for methodological reasons it was not possible to link particular complications to specific outcomes. Barker and Edwards (1967), using the Birmingham data on 50 000 children, achieved more focused results when they related verbal reasoning scores at 11 years of age to specified pregnancy and perinatal events. Five obstetric complications seemed to be associated with impaired verbal reasoning—a short gestation period, a prolonged gestation period (more than 41 weeks), toxaemia, occipito-posterior presentation, and delivery in an ambulance. Because the performance scores of children subjected to these events showed a unimodal distribution with no apparent bunching at the lower end of the scale, and because their scores were only slightly different from unaffected siblings, the authors concluded that it was 'unlikely that they [the complications] exert more than a small influence on the intellectual development of children exposed to them'. Use of factor analysis and multiple regression by Goldstein *et al.* (1976) on the Cattell DQ scores at one year of age in 322 infants showed significant effects of 'prematurity' (based on birth weight, gestational age, head circumference, and body length) and of 'delivery and related variables' (based primarily on type of birth and delivery, the use of drugs in pregnancy and delivery and Apgar score). Neligan *et al.* (1976) noted a possible association with antepartum haemorrhage, breech delivery, and fetal distress in labour in their data but discounted their intrinsic effect because their previous work had suggested that it became insignificant when associated biological and social factors were allowed for and because they knew of no other evidence suggesting a direct impact on performance.

There are other scattered findings in a rather unsatisfactory literature but the main conclusion must be that no fully convincing evidence has yet been produced showing the direct effect of obstetric factors on later functioning in LBW children.

Taking all the factors discussed in this section, our general conclusion is that the evidence points strongly to some direct influence of LBW and, particularly, of VLBW on a range of later competencies; that there is some evidence that children who were very-light-for-dates were also affected in their later functioning; but that there is little evidence of any substantial effect of pregnancy and delivery complications. All the studies suggest that socio-economic factors have a major and perhaps dominating influence on childhood functioning and that they may modify the effect of birth weight and gestation so that the correlation of birth weight and gestation with functioning will be weak in the upper social classes and strongest in the lower classes.

THE NEWBORN INFANT

During pregnancy the status of the fetus is assessed largely by inference from indirect observations. On delivery, detailed examination and measurement become possible, so that his condition can be determined with a much greater degree of precision. Formerly, the importance of this lay in indicating whether he was likely to live or die in the immediate neonatal period. However, the increased survival rate of infants and the consequent growth of interest in neurodevelopmental disability in later childhood promoted study of the newborn in the hope that features could be identified that would accurately predict future status. Attention has mainly been directed to the significance of neurological signs but the possible predictive value of other parameters has been the subject of extensive inquiry as well (e.g. Dawkins and MacGregor, 1965; Finnstrom, 1972; Cater, 1978). An infant's future may also depend on what happens to him in the perinatal period in terms of such factors as the effect of potentially injurious agents or the kind of care he receives: his eventual status may be modified by changing these variables and this too can be the basis of prediction.

The outcome for babies of low weight at birth may be expressed in terms of mortality rates or of the incidence of subsequent disability. Mortality is the easiest to ascertain, although there may be misunderstanding if it is not made clear whether rates are for first week deaths, neonatal deaths, infant deaths or total postnatal deaths. Major disability in survivors is a less clearly defined category, which usually includes manifest neurological and intellectual deficit, e.g. mental subnormality, cerebral palsy, serious loss of vision or hearing. Early studies laid emphasis on mortality and major disability but, with higher survival rates and a low level of major disability in survivors, minor disability has become increasingly used as a criterion of outcome, although it is ill-defined and often difficult to detect and to measure accurately. Indeed, to define it at all is to some extent artificial, since it merely represents one end of a continuum of disability and any cut-off point between major and minor will necessarily be arbitrary. Disabilities labelled 'minor' may nevertheless lead to serious degrees of handicap in affected children and it will not do to include them in the 'healthy' category of outcome simply because they are not easily measured (Stewart *et al.*, 1981).

The suggestion has been made on epidemiological grounds that neonatal intensive care methods may be more effective in preventing these lesser degrees of disability than the more severe forms, many of which have prenatal origins (*British Medical Journal*, 1979; Davies, 1980). On the other hand, Stewart and her colleagues (1981) say that the presence of minor handicaps appears often to be more closely related to adverse social and environmental factors than to perinatal events. It is apparent that much more information is needed on this subject and better ways of defining minor disability if the prediction of outcome is to be put on a more secure foundation.

We now proceed to consider briefly some of the features of the newborn infant which have been used as the basis for prediction.

Neurological status at birth

The physiology of the nervous system in infancy, especially reflex behaviour and responses to stimuli in the newborn period, was extensively explored in the early years of this century and then forgotten by all but a few (e.g. McGraw, 1943) until new interest was stimulated by the search for predictors of neurological outcome. André-Thomas and Saint-Anne Dargassies in Paris, Peiper in Leipzig, and Prechtl and his school in Groningen were pioneers in this field, opening the way to the intensive study of neonatal neurology of recent years. It is now clear that there is a generally increased risk of later disability amongst infants showing neurological abnormality in the newborn period, especially those with certain constellations of neurological signs (Nelson and Ellenberg, 1979; Volpe, 1979). Nevertheless, it is fair to say that the prognostic value of neurological signs in the individual infant has been less than was hoped for. This is partly because neurological status is influenced by the general condition of the infant at birth and represents the sum of many intrinsic and extraneous elements, not all of which have persisting effects, and partly because the developing brain in the postnatal period is subject to a wide variety of environmental influences whch may affect later function (Beintema, 1968; Littman and Parmelee, 1978). Prediction may be more reliable if neurological assessment is combined with other indices, such as signs of perinatal asphyxia and

EEG abnormalities (Scheiner, 1980). Moreover, Prechtl's recent emphasis on optimal and suboptimal neurological status at birth, rather than overt abnormality, holds out promise of greater predictive capability (Prechtl, 1977; Njiokiktjien and Kurver, 1980). Finally, there is some evidence that neurological examination can more reliably forecast normality than abnormality, on which most attention has hitherto been focused (Dennis, 1978).

Apart from its possible role in prediction, evaluation of the neonatal nervous system has proved useful in estimating the developmental stage attained at birth and has been incorporated into clinical practice for this purpose. Precise details of neurological testing and interpretation have been published by Saint-Anne Dargassies (1974) and Prechtl (1977), while many workers have reported shortened modified systems of neurological examination of the newborn for routine use in clinical practice (e.g. Robinson, 1966; Koenigsberger, 1966; Finnstrom, 1971). More recent interest has centred on a wider assessment of neonatal behaviour as a possible predictor of future personality and social as well as neuromuscular development (Brazelton, 1973).

External physical characteristics

The general appearance of an infant born many weeks early is very different from that of the infant born at term, apart from the disparity in size. The features which distinguish the two have been used by clinicians for many years as an indication of gestational age but their observations lacked precision until numerical values could be assigned to the individual physical signs. In the early 1960s, joint research studies between Aberdeen and Newcastle-upon-Tyne defined some of the more important characteristics and developed a scoring system based on these definitions (Mitchell and Farr, 1965; Farr et al., 1966a and b). At about the same time other workers, notably Usher in Montreal, were thinking along similar lines (Usher et al., 1966). Since then many have applied these measurements in research and clinical practice, modifying them in various ways to suit particular purposes (e.g. Parkin et al., 1976; Latis et al., 1981). Other workers have selected certain neurological and physical characteristics and combined them, sometimes with anthropometric and other measurements, into composite scoring systems which may in some circumstances give more accurate estimates of gestational age at birth than either set of characteristics on its own (Dubowitz et al., 1970).

The importance of determining the stage of maturation reached at the time of birth, and of inferring from that the infant's gestational age, lies in the implications for ultimate outcome and in the possibility of predicting it, since this depends on the ability to relate gestational age to birth weight as precisely as possible. Earlier studies of low weight at birth did not take gestational age into account and even recent work sometimes ignores differences between babies born early and babies who are light-for-dates or bases the assessment of gestational age on obstetric criteria—notoriously fallacious—without reference to the condition of the infant at birth. Yet comparisons between groups of infants must take account of the relationship between duration of pregnancy and fetal growth if the significance of such factors as socio-economic background, quality of neonatal care, postnatal health, and loss from follow-up is to be properly evaluated (Kiely and Paneth, 1981).

Perinatal asphyxia

Birth requires the infant to make rapid and radical adjustments, not only to the external world but also to changes in his internal milieu consequent on separation from the placenta. Healthy infants born at term make these adaptations relatively easily but those born early or poorly grown have greater difficulties. The most pressing need is to stabilize the pattern of blood gases and acid/base balance, which has been disturbed by the events of birth to show lower oxygen levels, increased carbon dioxide and acidaemia—the changes collectively known as asphyxial. Perinatal asphyxia is a recognized antecedent of neurological disability but the exact causal relationship has not been established and some severely asphyxiated infants apparently escape all damage (Scott, 1976; Thomson et al., 1977; de Souza and Richards, 1978). The degree and duration of asphyxia in the newborn infant have therefore been much studied as possible indicators of subsequent abnormality. The LBW infant is especially at risk but it has proved difficult to separate the effects of asphyxia from those of immaturity, method of delivery, biochemical disturbance, and neonatal illness, since these are all closely interrelated. The use of multiple criteria of asphyxia, together with the infant's response to it, may increase the reliability with which developmental sequelae can be predicted (Scheiner, 1980) but so far results have been inconclusive. As a result of this uncertainty, there is continuing controversy about the consequences of asphyxia at birth for the future development of the child.

Quality of care

Clarification of the role of asphyxia is rendered more difficult by constantly changing fashions in neonatal care. Some therapeutic measures, such as delayed feeding and misuse of oxygen, have themselves caused disability, especially in children who were of low weight at birth (Davies, 1978). Such infants are especially vulnerable to nutritional deprivation and therefore the nature of their feeding in the newborn period may have a bearing on their ultimate neurological status (Davies and Evans, 1978). The extensive use of mechanical ventilation in recent years has led to fears that babies who would have died might survive with neurological damage, and there is evidence that this may sometimes be the case (Marriage and Davies, 1977). On the other hand, survivors who have been ventilated under carefully controlled conditions have shown no such sequelae (Dinwiddie *et al.*, 1974). Rapid advances in intensive neonatal care and the widespread and sometimes indiscriminate adoption of new methods do carry risks of increasing the survival rate of brain-damaged babies (Kitchen *et al.*, 1979) though this may be offset by the intact survival of other infants who might have survived with neurological disability had they not been treated by the new techniques. A review by Paneth and his colleagues (1981) makes it clear that declining mortality rates amongst LBW infants must be accompanied by an even greater rate of decline in neurological impairment amongst the survivors if the eventual prevalence of handicap is not to be increased. There is much evidence that the introduction of modern neonatal intensive care methods has been accompanied by substantial increases in survival rates (Thompson and Reynolds, 1977). It is therefore reassuring to learn that, in a long-term follow-up of LBW infants, comparing two groups born 15 years apart during which management in the neonatal period had changed considerably, Drillien and her colleagues (1980) concluded that, despite improvement in the survival rate, the incidence of handicap among survivors had not increased.

While it is tempting to attribute improvements in outcome to advances in intensive care, the causal relationship has not been firmly established and other trends have to be taken into account, such as changes in obstetric practice, in the social and economic environment, and in the characteristics of infants of similar birth weight. Some of the difficulties in interpretation are illustrated by reports on the outcome for infants of very low birth weight (VLBW), on which much attention has recently been focused. Stewart and her colleagues (1981) have summarized the results of 16 studies which considered the outcome for infants weighing up to 1500 g at birth. Most workers define VLBW in this way though 2000 g and less may be chosen by some and occasionally other ranges, such as 501 to 1250 or 1500 g. With increasing intensity of management of such VLBW infants, increased survival rates and diminished disability rates in survivors have been recorded in many hospitals (e.g. Rawlings *et al.*, 1971; Stewart and Reynolds, 1974; Pape *et al.*, 1978; Westgren *et al.*, 1982; Hirata *et al.*, 1983). These reports must be interpreted with caution, however, for they are not always based on total population studies and they represent the achievements of the best units rather than the average.

One important study which considered all VLBW infants born in a specified geographical area is that by Stanley and Alberman (1978). They reported on 692 live-born infants of 2000 g or less, representing 98 per cent of all those born in three south-east London boroughs in a three-year period between 1970 and 1973. After excluding 7 infants with lethal congenital malformations, the neonatal mortality rate was 303.5 per 1000 live births: there were no significant associations between neonatal mortality and maternal age, social class, race, marital status or parity. Mortality was significantly higher when there was a history of a previous stillbirth, neonatal death or abortion. The infants were cared for in different hospital units and the neonatal mortality rate for infants in the best equipped and staffed unit was significantly lower than that for comparable infants nursed in the unit with the poorest facilities. This and other reports (e.g. Davies and Stewart, 1975; Franco and Andrews, 1977; Chiswick *et al.*, 1979; Vohr and Hack, 1982; Horwood *et al.*, 1982) suggest that modern intensive care methods have improved the outlook for VLBW infants.

Claims for the efficacy of intensive care have not gone unchallenged. Steiner and his colleagues (1980) reported the outcome for 293 infants weighing from 501 to 1500 g at birth and born in a geographically defined area in England. In the hospital unit where they were cared for, standards of nursing care and record-keeping were said to be consistently high, medical care to be conscientious but almost exclusively of a non-interventionist type, and policy to have remained unchanged throughout the period in question. Of the 293 infants, 154 died in the neonatal period (52.6 per cent) and there were 137 long-term survivors, of whom 131 were seen between ages 6 and 16 years. Of these, 18 had major disabilities and 31 minor ones (6.1 and 10.5 per cent respectively of the total cohort). These results are compared by the authors with those from hospital units where high standards of modern intensive care are practised. For example, Hammersmith Hospital, London, with a neonatal mortality rate of 58.5 per cent and rates for major and minor disability of 5.3 and 5.6 per cent, respectively: and University College Hospital, London, with 44.7 per cent for neonatal mortality and 4.6 per cent for major disability. The authors conclude that scientific and highly skilled medical intervention in the years under discussion made little impact on the outcome for infants of very low birth weight. Subsequent correspondence in the *British Medical Journal* (e.g. Reynolds, 1980; Reynolds and Stewart, 1980; Houlsby and Lloyd, 1980; Dunn and Speidel, 1980; Hughes-Davies, 1981) revealed considerable differences of opinion on the interpretation of these findings and on the validity of the conclusion, illustrating the difficulty of making comparisons between uncontrolled series of data with multiple variables, both recognized and unrecognized.

Modern methods of intensive care of infants are based on scientific study, much of it in animals, and future advances must surely rest on such solid foundations rather than on an intuitive approach to care, however solicitous. Nobody who has practical experience in neonatal hospital units would suggest that intensive methods are a substitute for careful and conscientious nursing, for both are essential parts of a comprehensive programme. Equally none would deny that new techniques have to be tried out in practice and that not all will prove to be wholly beneficial. As methods become established, so their limitations are recognized and their hazards eliminated, with consequent improvement in results. With this continually changing pattern, it becomes impossible to make valid predictions on the basis of quality of care alone and in any case this is likely to have changed before results become known.

The essential components of good care are careful observation, accurate measurement of deviations from the physiological norms, and prompt action to correct such deviations before they can affect the infant adversely. Given these basic elements, controlled evaluation of new techniques must continue if outcome is to be further improved. When less than one third of VLBW infants born alive survive undamaged, the results are rightly considered disastrous (Reynolds, 1980). Whether the increase in the proportion of undamaged survivors to over half by the late 1970s (Stewart *et al.*, 1981) is the result of improved management or not, the possibility that it is justifies the call for more and better distribution of modern neonatal care facilities. It is important, however, that further development is controlled and that advanced equipment is not indiscriminately provided in hospitals without the skilled staff to use it properly.

The lowering of mortality in LBW (and especially VLBW) babies and improved methods of neonatal care may have changed the probability of damage in surviving children. However, these developments in neonatal medicine could have conflicting implications. Better neonatal care may have prevented certain sequelae occurring at earlier periods. On the other hand, it could have ensured the survival of babies with residual damage. From the research viewpoint, this means that studies conducted at different times during the last two decades might each reach different, but accurate, conclusions. It also indicates that, even more than previously, it is necessary to examine separately the results for babies falling into different categories of LBW.

POSTNATAL INFLUENCES

Every claim in the literature for a direct causative relationship between pregnancy and perinatal events and the child's subsequent level of performance is examined with cautious scepticism as a possible artefact stemming from the hidden operation of the child's postnatal experiences. As we have seen from the preceding review, apparently strong correlations have frequently been reduced to insignificance when allowance has been made for associated social and biological factors of largely postnatal origin. Illsley (1967) reviewed in detail the theoretical and methodological problems inherent in the interpretation of such correlations, giving examples of alternative models of explanation for simple asociations between social and biological factors and between prenatal and postnatal influences.

Low weight at birth and disability in childhood each have multi-factorial origins involving varying combinations of genetic, biological, and social factors which interact and may modify one another. In attempting to isolate a causal connection, we are abstracting both the presumed cause and the presumed outcome from a long process of interaction of influences which militates against a unifactorial explanation. A simplified representation of these interacting in-

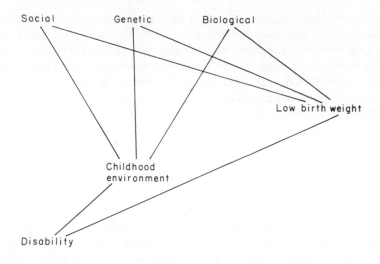

Figure 2.1   Parental background.

fluences is shown in Figure 2.1. It portrays LBW as the outcome of interacting parental characteristics whose relative weightings are speculative for LBW as a population category and *a fortiori* more speculative for the individual birth. Other manifestations of those same parental/family characteristics, again combined with varying weightings, have a direct influence upon the child's postnatal environment. Our analytical problem is to determine whether a specific disability is mediated through LBW alone, through the child's environment alone, or through a combination of both. A direct link between parental characteristics, childhood environment, and disability (ignoring LBW) is known to exist because it occurs in children across the full range of birth weights. The model, as drawn, is of course incomplete in that we could postulate direct links between parental (e.g. genetic) characteristics and a specific disability.

No study has been able to document precisely the composition of each of these interacting influences. Parental characteristics, for example, are usually inferred from a few proxy indicators, such as the father's occupation and the mother's height. More important, very few studies have attempted to observe and document in any depth the socio-cultural experiences of children in the family, the school, and the neighbourhood. Rather than attempt direct study of the postnatal environment, most investigators have attempted to eliminate differences in that environment by using a control group matched for a variety of social factors at the time of pregnancy or birth (i.e. before the commencement of the postnatal period). The underlying rationale, that prenatal social matching ensures matching of the postnatal environment, predicates the use of several unjustified assumptions. First, that those aspects of maternal social experience relevant to pregnancy and delivery are equally relevant to the process of child development and, second, that there is no inter-generational change in social status and social behaviour. Following his own experience of a matched control study of premature children, Douglas (1960) remarks on the misleading results likely to follow from the first assumption. Illsley (1980), in a study of the social and reproductive correlates of inter- and intra-generational social mobility, shows quite marked variations within maternal social classes identified at first pregnancy in factors relating to the upbringing and development of their children. The use of sibling comparisons (Barker, 1966; McKeown, 1970) avoids this assumption but has the corresponding defect that it obviates the necessity of studying the postnatal environment because its relevance to child development has been eliminated in order to concentrate on birth weight itself. Except in a few studies, the events occurring between departure from the maternity hospital and the time of outcome assessment have been ignored. The omission is understandable, both on the grounds that most studies have been organized by hospital-based medical research workers and because direct observation of the social environment over a period of years is extremely time-consuming of resources.

The number of studies deploying data about pregnancy, neonatal status, and even minimal information about the postnatal period, and relating these data to measures of outcome is consequently very small indeed. Douglas and co-workers (Douglas and Blomfield, 1958; Douglas, 1960; Douglas and Gear, 1976) followed up a cohort of LBW children born in 1946 and reported on their development at the ages of 5 and 15. While he used a matched control group, he did examine the differential experience of LBW and control children on several dimensions. In 1958 he reported: an excess of hospital admissions up to the age of 2 years due primarily to lower respiratory infections; small weight and stature at age 4; and low scores on tests of reading, vocabulary, and mental ability. Similar results on these tests were found at age 11 accompanied by other strong evidence of lower educational achievement. These results prompted Douglas to examine the efficiency of his matching criteria and he found that the parents of the LBW children ranked lower than the controls on their class and educational background and on assessments previously made by health visitors of standards of care and management and of interest in the child's school progress; he concluded that these factors, rather than birth weight, accounted for the differential achievement of his groups. Subsequent study of an alternative sample of the same children, but excluding those between 2000 and 2500 g, found no significant differences in mental and physical handicap or test performance. These results are puzzling in view of Douglas' earlier demonstration of the incompleteness of matching and of his comment in the later article that there was likely to be increasing social differentiation between experimental and control groups over time. Sameroff and Chandler (1975) quote many other instances of early differences in functioning which become attenuated at later ages.

The other major British longitudinal study (Davie *et al.*, 1972) reports very substantial differences between social classes in IQ, reading and arithmetic attainment, and a range of behavioural items, and we have already seen above that social class and family size contributed much more strongly to these differences than birth weight or maternal height. Unfortunately, no analysis was made of the relationship of birth weight and performance to the very large number of class-related attitudes, values, and aspects of living conditions and behaviour collected during the course of the survey. The study of Neligan *et al.* (1976) was interesting in its identification of maternal care as a major influence on development but again its day-to-day meaning was not investigated.

The literature contains other partial evidence about the different postnatal environments of LBW children compared with children who were heavier at birth. This literature was systematically reviewed by Birch and Gussow (1970) and the quotation from their review reproduced above, which referred to the disadvantaged children and not specifically to LBW children, adequately sums up the state of present knowledge. It is, however, a composite statement, bringing together well-proven facts, tendencies, and speculations, and one which creates a plausible pattern through inferential reasoning. Specific relationships and their place in the presumed pattern still need testing.

The dearth of literature focusing specifically upon postnatal experience as a mediator between birth weight and childhood functioning means that we have to rely upon the general literature on child development to interpret the every-day experiential meaning of general parameters known to be associated with being small at birth, e.g. social class, family size, maternal care, and known also to be causally related to the types of disability documented in studies of LBW children. These parameters properly belong to a monograph on child development and are too numerous and complex to be reviewed in this chapter. The essential point for future research is that they consist of innumerable daily interactions of the child with his cultural, psychological, and physical environment and cannot be captured by the use of a few general indicators based not on his actual experience but on the characteristics of heterogeneous aggregates such as lower social classes or large families.

THE ASSESSMENT OF ABILITIES, ATTRIBUTES, AND BEHAVIOUR

The total literature on the later characteristics of LBW infants compared with heavier infants records a multitude of deficits in LBW children across a wide range of indicators of physiological, neurological, temperamental, behavioural, and intellectual functioning. Measurements have been carried out by different investigators, at different ages, using a variety of tests and indicators. With samples of different size and composition, studied at different ages and in different contexts, there are inevitably some discrepancies and disagreements on particular items. On the whole, however, there is a remarkable degree of consistency. The most comprehensive battery of measurements was carried out by Neligan and his colleagues (1976) on 7-year-old children. Summing up their results, these authors described 'a picture which is clear and consistent' and in particular stated:

> The children in one or both of our two extreme abnormal groups (short gestation and very light-for-dates) have 'worse' scores than those in the control group (a random sample of births from which short-gestation and light-for-dates infants were excluded) in every single instance where a direct comparison can be made, and the differences are statistically significant. This applies not only to the total scores for complete tests, but also to every individual test.

It was not our purpose in this study to question or duplicate such widely demonstrated findings. Our purpose was to understand the contexts in which and the processes by which these differences arose and specifically to examine the degree to which differences arose, not from birth weight itself but from the different social backgrounds of LBW and heavier children. We therefore used a more selected set of measurements and assessments of children's physical status and performance at the 10-year follow-up viz. anthropometric characteristics, signs of neurological functioning obtained by medical examination and by scores on the Bender-Gestalt test, and intellectual abilities based on the WISC test and sub-tests. These measurements and assessments are described in the relevant chapters elsewhere in this book. At this stage we merely wish to remark on some general features of the data which are important for interpretative purposes.

The first point relates to the stages in the child's history at which these data were obtained. Data on the child relate to three points in time—at birth, at 10 months, and at 10 years. Data on the parents and on the social environment of the child were collected either during pregnancy or in the days following the birth when the mother was still in hospital. The child's environment therefore was not directly studied but must be inferred from the social circumstances of the parents around the time of the child's birth and from opinions, attitudes, and aspects of parental behaviour elicited from the mother at that time. There is therefore a long period between the time of these observations and the time of assessment at follow-up. This obviously creates problems of interpretation. Some of the studies quoted above suffer from a similar deficiency, while others (e.g. Neligan, 1976 and Davie et al., 1972) collected social information at the point of assessment. All studies suffer from the common deficiency that little or no information was collected in the interval between birth and assessment (often many years after birth).

The second and related point concerns the use of direct and indirect indicators. Clinical interest in the child and the desire to establish as clearly as possible the specific abilities and deficits of each child give most of the follow-up studies a characteristic pattern. Whatever the age of measurement, it is usual for each child to be assessed individually. Thus in most studies we have direct data for each child on some of the clinical features of intra-uterine experience and delivery and a variety of measures of intellectual performance (typically IQ scores and measures of reading ability), neurological and psychiatric status, and anthropometric characteristics.

Unfortunately, other data frequently used as interpretative material cannot be gathered by direct measurement and observation. Therefore investigators are forced to use general indicators, known to be related to the required characteristic but involving approximation and second-hand reports or judgments. The most obvious example is 'social class'. This variable is used as a substitute for something much more complex. Ideally we would like to know for each child how the child's development is affected by his daily interaction with and experience of his physical, social, intellectual, and emotional environment. A child's dietary experience between birth and measurement at age 7 to 10 years consists of a multitude of events, hour by hour and day by day, the input of food in both quantity and quality varying across the years and varying between families. If data are available (and this is very rare), they are based upon mothers' accounts taken at a point in time and summated subjectively by the interviewer. There are, of course, certain consistencies in family behaviour but our measurements can only be a poor reflection of reality. Neligan's very important variable 'the mother's care of the child', was obtained by these methods and, although the interviewers were obviously perceptive, the indicator can only be a gross approximation to the daily physical, verbal, and emotional exchanges between the mother and child over many years, some of which may have been mutually contradictory, e.g. the kind of regime which provides physical care, warmth, and nutrition but which represses emotional feeling or intellectual exploration. When so much emphasis is placed upon early bonding, on affective behaviour, and on the role of other family members in healthy child-rearing, a single judgment made on the basis of a limited observation seems inadequate to the task. Intellectual growth is a complex composite of many experiences; of stimulation and restrictiveness; of listening to, watching or participating in many verbal and visual interactions; of formal education, spontaneous reading, and informal learning. Obviously, crude indicators based on years at school or teachers' reports can hardly encapsulate a tiny fraction of the formative influences. Social class in the absence of other material is intended to summarize all these experiences and many others derived from contact with and responses to the behaviour, attitudes, and values of adult and peer groups, as well as the physical/biological factors of housing, warmth, sickness, exercise, etc. We know from innumerable studies and, particularly, from studies of social mobility that variations within classes are sometimes as large as variations across classes and that many persons in lower class backgrounds acquire middle class attributes; yet investigators frequently treat 'social class' based on the father's occupational group (not his personal characteristics or even his precise occupation) as a substitute for life experience. The population is often divided into 2 or 3 class groups and data analysed within them as if social variation had thus been eliminated.

We draw this to the reader's attention because, faute de mieux, we shall often do the same and because it brings great interpretative problems. An analysis of maternal height against child's height will be based on direct measurement of each of the individuals analysed. A comparison of the child's Wechsler score against a Bender score, for all the difficulties of interpretation, will say something direct about the child's performance on two tests. An analysis of the child's parental social class against the teacher's rating of his social behaviour at school translated into these other variables is rather like comparing the average IQ of the child's school against the school nurse's estimate of neurological functioning.

The point has significance for the strength of relationships revealed by correlation coefficients or multiple regression. Most of the indirect variables are low in validity and have a great scatter round the mean. If social class is shown to have statistical significance in a regression equation alongside directly measured characteristics, it indicates the presence of some very strong influence which is able partially to shine through gross contamination. The same point has relevance for matching by social class—it is one of the best available measures but it cannot achieve the social equivalence of groups.

A similar qualification and caution must be applied to the cross-tabulation of two indirect variables against one of the child's measured attributes. If, for example, we find a strong relationship between the father's social class and the child's IQ and wish to take the analysis a stage further by looking at the joint relationship of father's and mother's occupational class against IQ, we certainly achieve greater discrimination. Within a given father's occupational class we shall find clear and ordered differences of IQ according to the mother's occupational class. This does not say anything directly about the mother's contribution to the child's intellectual development. Instead it breaks down the class into smaller and more homogeneous groups, a process which might equally well be achieved by the use of other variables unrelated to the mother, e.g. housing tenure. We may infer something extra about the children's environments by knowing, for example, that some children of skilled workers have mothers with professional qualifications while others have unskilled mothers. However, it would be dangerous to conclude that the extra discrimination derives from the mother's personal qualities and contribution rather than from a composite family influence.

CONCLUSION

It is clear that the relationship between low weight at birth and ultimate outcome for the infant is extremely complex. It is influenced not only by the genetic endowment of the child and the nature and intensity of perinatal events, but also by the degree of interaction with the postnatal environment—such features as attacks by infective and other noxious agents or the quality of care and protection given—and the extent of compensation which the child can make for disability originating in earlier life. In a minority of instances prenatal or perinatal abnormality is so great that subsequent disability can confidently be predicted; in many more the association is not as obvious and indeed may be so influenced by chance happenings or by planned intervention that the expected outcome does not materialize. It is not surprising therefore that there is considerable uncertainty about causal relationships, not least because the quality of recorded observation is often inadequate and subsequent follow-up is discontinuous. One of the main purposes of the present study was to reduce this uncertainty by establishing for an unselected population of LBW infants a corpus of detailed, carefully recorded observations about the events surrounding birth, and by amassing data of comparable reliability about the environment into which the child was born and into which he would grow up. With such basic information, the status of the child in later life—in this case at the age of ten years—could more confidently be related to his antecedents in the light of his inborn characteristics and major life events during the intervening period.

Since the data which might be recorded about a child between fetal life and a postnatal age of ten years are almost infinite, decisions had to be made at the planning stage about the items to be observed or measured. The temptation to accumulate large masses of information on the grounds that it might be relevant was rejected in favour of the careful observation and recording of a relatively small number of items which might be expected to influence outcome on grounds of existing knowledge or reasonable supposition. Thus, in addition to background social and obstetric data, information was gathered about the infant's weight, gestational age, and condition at birth; his neurological status, physical characteristics and biochemical deviations from normal in the first few days; and his postnatal progress. The subsequent chapters are largely concerned with relating these findings to the later outcome for the child and especially with attempts to identify the differential influences of low weight at birth and the social environment. The extent to which we have been successful in achieving these objectives is considered in Chapters 9 and 10.

Chapter 3

The Design and Methods of the Study

M. RUSSELL, B. THOMPSON, AND M. SAMPHIER

THE POPULATION

The study sample and the controls were drawn from the population of Aberdeen city and suburbs, which in 1969–70, when the study children were born, covered an area of nearly 20 square miles (51 square kilometres) between the rivers Don and Dee, and to the south of the Dee, on the north–east coast of Scotland. Aberdeen was then the fourth largest city in Scotland and the principal seaport of the north–east, acting as its administrative, commercial, educational, and industrial focus. Up to that time the city had a relatively stable population, partly due to its geographical isolation (the two nearest large towns are Dundee, 70 miles (112 km) to the south, and Inverness, 100 miles (160 km) to the north–west) and partly due to the ease of obtaining employment locally (Illsley *et al.*, 1963). After 1970 rapid changes were to accompany the increasing commercial and industrial activity associated with the exploration for and production of North Sea oil (Grampian Regional Council, 1980). In 1971, the nearest national census year to the sample selection period, the city population was 182 071 and the rate of unemployment in the population aged 15 and over was only 3.6 per cent (1971 National Census—county of Aberdeen city). The major industries included fishing, granite dressing and polishing, paper manufacture, shipbuilding and engineering, textiles, knitting and clothing manufacture, and food processing. Aberdeen was also the commercial and administrative centre for the agricultural hinterland. In addition, employment was offered by the university, research institutes, colleges, health board, and local council.

For the purposes of a follow-up study, the population available had the advantage of being geographically and economically stable and ethnically homogeneous. The location and characteristics of Aberdeen provided opportunities for the development of a comprehensive maternity service and records system by collaboration between hospital and local government authorities. Since 1948, Aberdeen Maternity Hospital has maintained records, including medical, obstetric and social data, of all births, whether in hospital, in the NHS domiciliary service or in private practice, occurring to women resident in the defined geographical area of Aberdeen city and immediate suburbs (now known as Aberdeen District, estimated population 220 000 in the late 1970s). A computerized obstetric data bank has recently been established retrospectively to 1948 and is being continuously maintained (Samphier and Thompson, 1981). Although the present study is based on hospital births only, these accounted for over 98 per cent of the deliveries to residents of Aberdeen city and suburbs in the period 1969–70.

SELECTION AND MATCHING FOR THE SAMPLE

Matching criteria

On broad epidemiological criteria we already knew a good deal about how LBW and heavier babies differed in the social characteristics of their parents. The influence of social class and birth weight on later intellectual functioning is statistically well established, but the problem remaining was to disentangle the specific contributions of each. In considering the later development and functioning of LBW infants, various hypotheses have emphasized: 1. the influence of prenatal factors; 2. the contribution of social background and styles of living; 3. the genetic component. This dictated the choice of a controlled study in which major confounding variables could be excluded by research design and in which other factors could be studied in detail on a relatively small sample. The choice of matching variables was necessarily limited by the range of data collected routinely for each birth. Three matching variables—the husband's social class, the child's sex, and his ordinal position in the family—were chosen because of their direct and indirect influence upon the child's social environment. With two populations comparable in these respects it would be possible to see more clearly the role of other social influences on the relationship between birth weight and functioning. The two remaining variables used for matching—maternal height and smoking habits—were chosen because of their known relationship to the aetiology of birth weight and because they each had an additional social significance. Average birth weight varies directly with maternal height, and failure to control for height would have produced unmanageable comparisons between small children of small mothers and large children of taller mothers. Control for height would make it possible systematically to ask how small and larger babies of mothers of similar height differed from each other and also to look for differences between the children of mothers of different height. Maternal height also varies with social class and its use for matching gives additional socio-economic control. Similarly, the inclusion of smoking reduces the aetiological heterogeneity of sample and control cases, but strengthens socio-economic matching in that smoking is inversely related to parental social class.

To achieve a further degree of homogeneity between sample and control groups, the study population was drawn entirely from legitimate singleton babies born to residents of Aberdeen city and its immediate suburbs over a defined period.

Exclusions from the sample

Because of the difficulty in matching a relatively small number of illegitimate LBW infants with illegitimate controls who share all the previously specified matching criteria, and because of the difficulties involved in following up illegitimate children, who often undergo changes in name and address during their early years, these were excluded from the sample. Multiple births were also excluded because their aetiology and prognosis are known to be different from those of singleton births, and many of the hypotheses explored in this study would only be applicable to singletons.

In addition to these two main categories, births were excluded if the families were in excessively mobile occupations, e.g. the Armed Forces, due to the difficulty in following up their children, or if the families were non-Caucasian, due to the problems in finding controls matched on five criteria in addition to race, in an almost totally Caucasian population (1971 National Census—county of Aberdeen city). Children of the staff associated with the project were excluded, in the interests of maintaining confidentiality, and births to women for whom social class could not be adequately defined, e.g. women married to students, were also excluded.

Selection of the LBW study sample

Bearing these considerations in mind, the study sample was a one-year cohort of LBW babies surviving the neonatal period, and born in Aberdeen Maternity Hospital during the period 1st July 1969 to 30th June 1970, to mothers residing in the city and suburbs of Aberdeen. Table 3.1 shows that there were 3007 births in that year of which 74 (2.4 per cent) were twins: 35 of these were LBW, accounting for 13.8 per cent of the 254 LBW babies. Of the 219 LBW singletons, 21 were stillborn and 21 died within 28 days. The remaining 177 LBW singletons were therefore 'at risk' to selection for the study.

Table 3.2 shows that, after the exclusions described above, the study sample

Table 3.1 LBW and total births July 1969–June 1970

	Singletons			Twins			All births		
Outcome	LBW	Total	% LBW	LBW	Total	% LBW	LBW	Total	% LBW
Stillbirths	21	29	72.4	—	—	—	21	29	72.4
Neonatal deaths	21	31	67.7	4	5	80.0	25	36	69.4
Survivors	177	2873	6.2	31	69	44.9	208	2942	7.1
Total	219	2933	7.5	35	74	47.3	254	3007	8.5

Table 3.2 The total population of births from which the LBW and control samples were taken

Birth weight period	2500 g or less: July 1969–June 1970		Over 2500 g: July 1969–December 1970	
	No.	%	No.	%
Singleton				
Survivor				
Study population	145[5]	57.1	149[1]*	3.5*
Refused	1	0.4	7	0.2
Missed	8	3.2	0	0
Excluded	12†	4.7	3720	88.1
Illegitimate	11	4.3	268	6.4
Total	177	69.7	4144	98.2
Death				
Stillborn	21	8.3	9	0.2
In first month	21	8.3	14	0.3
Total	42	16.6	23	0.5
Twin				
Survivor				
Legitimate	29	11.4	53	1.3
Illegitimate	2	0.8	0	0
Total	31	12.2	53	1.3
Death				
Stillbirth	0	0	0	0
In first month	4	1.5	0	0
Total	4	1.5	0	0
All births	254	100.0	4220	100.0

[1], [5] Illegitimate according to subsequent sociological interview.

* Includes the controls of the 4 additional LBW babies born to upper social class primigravidae

† Excluded as a member of staff, known to be leaving Aberdeen, or of unclassifiable social class, or on grounds of ethnic origin.

totalled 145 of the 166 legitimate singleton LBW infants resident in the city and suburbs of Aberdeen.

The sample was augmented to 149 babies by a further 4 LBW infants selected after the one-year period, in order to increase the proportion of infants whose mothers were upper social class primigravidae, since these had proved the most difficult subjects to enlist, due to the scarcity of LBW babies born to upper social class women.

A sub-sample of 32 families was interviewed again 10 months later by the sociologist in order to explore more fully the effects of contrasting environmental circumstances on the early development of these babies. This sub-sample was composed of the families in the extreme social classes who had no previous surviving children.

Selection of the controls and matching procedures

Each LBW baby was matched with the next occurring legitimate singleton baby of birth weight more than 2500 g, drawn from the same population of Caucasian parents resident in the city or suburbs of Aberdeen, on five characteristics: the baby's sex and ordinal position in the family, and maternal smoking, social class, and height. Due to the difficulty in matching on five separate criteria, the time period for selecting controls had to be extended by 6 months to 31 December 1970. This extended time accounts for the difference between the total number of births in Tables 3.1 and 3.2. Of the controls selected, 7 mothers refused to allow their babies to be included in the study; in these instances, the next infant delivered with suitable matching characteristics was enrolled as the control.

Table 3.3 gives the percentage of LBW/control pairs for which exact matching was achieved.

1. The LBW and control groups were exactly matched for sex, with 74 boys and 75 girls in each.
2. The baby's ordinal position in the family was taken as 1, 2, 3 or 4 + and on this basis 97 per cent of pairs were matched. Table 3.4 shows that in both

Table 3.3 Success in matching LBW/control pairs on different criteria

| Criterion | No. of pairs | | Per cent matched |
	Matched	Not matched	
1. Sex of baby	149	—	100
2. Ordinal position in family	145	4	97
3. Smoking: ever/never	140	9	94
4. Social class-group	131	18	88
5. Maternal height within 5 cm	116	33	78

Table 3.4 Child's ordinal number in the family

Ordinal number	LBW	(%)	Controls	(%)
1	78	(52.3)	79	(53.0)
2	36	(24.2)	39	(26.2)
3	26	(17.4)	22	(14.7)
4+	9	(6.1)	9	(6.1)
Total	149	(100.0)	149	(100.0)

$\chi^2 = 0.46$, d.f. $= 3, p = 0.93$.

groups over half the babies would be either an only child or the eldest in their family whereas 6 per cent already had at least 3 older siblings.

3. Due to difficulty in obtaining reliable information about the number of cigarettes smoked at a particular time or about smoking behaviour during pregnancy, and to the necessity for close matching on the other four variables, the women were simply divided into those who were smokers and those who were non-smokers at the time of their first visit to the antenatal clinic. It was most difficult to find suitable controls who were smokers and in the end there were 4 more LBW babies than controls whose mothers smoked. It may be noted that over one-third of the pairs were non-smokers (Table 3.5).

Table 3.5 Maternal smoking at the first visit to the antenatal clinic

Smoked	LBW	(%)	Controls	(%)
No	53	(35.6)	57	(38.3)
Yes	96	(64.4)	92	(61.7)
Total	149	(100.0)	149	(100.0)

$\chi^2 = 0.13$, d.f. $= 1, p = 0.72$.

4. Social class was derived from the occupation of the father and based on the Registrar General's Classification of Occupations 1960, divided as follows:

Social Class   I   Professional
               II   Managerial/executive/technical } Non-manual
               IIIa Other white collar

               IIIb Skilled manual   Skilled manual

               IV   Semi-skilled   } Other manual
               V   Unskilled manual

In the beginning the six social class groups were used in matching but it soon became obvious that this was not feasible within the limits of the study and therefore matching based on three broad occupational groups—non-manual, skilled manual, and other manual—was permitted when unavoidable. Accurate matching was achieved in 75.8 per cent of pairs using the six social classes but was increased to 87.9 per cent of pairs when only the three occupational groups were considered. Nevertheless 18 (12.1 per cent) LBW babies were necessarily paired with controls in other occupational groups. Table 3.6 shows that there were equal numbers of LBW and control babies whose fathers were in non-manual occupations, but 4 more LBW than control babies had fathers in the least skilled manual occupations ('other manual').

Table 3.6 Social class—derived from husband's occupation

Social Class		LBW	(%)	Controls	(%)
I	⎫	9	(6.0)	10	(6.7)
II	⎬ Non-	14	(9.4)	15	(10.1)
IIIa	⎭ manual	12	(8.1)	10	(6.7)
IIIb	Skilled manual	52	(34.9)	56	(37.6)
IV	⎫ Other	26	(17.4)	24	(16.1)
V	⎬ manual	36	(24.2)	34	(22.8)
Total		149	(100.0)	149	(100.0)

$\chi^2 = 0.55$, d.f. $= 5$, $p = 0.99$.

5. Initially, matching for maternal height was based on three categories relevant to the Aberdeen population and used extensively in obstetric practice and research:

'Small': 154 cm or less ($<5'\ 1''$)
'Medium': 155 cm to 162 cm ($5'\ 1'' - 5'\ 4''$)
'Tall': 163 cm and over ($>5'4''$)

In the early stages of matching, these categories were rigidly adhered to but as the selection of controls progressed it became apparent that within the categories of 'small' and 'tall' it was possible to have fairly large differences between the heights of the study sample and their controls. To obviate this, these categories were replaced by a specification that controls should be within 5 cm (2'') of their study counterparts.

Table 3.7 shows that there was an excess of 16 more LBW mothers in the 'small' group, and 4 more control mothers in the 'tall' group.

When the 5 cm difference in height between LBW and controls was applied, 33 pairs (22.2 per cent) were outside this limit, some of the controls in

Table 3.7 Maternal height

Height group	LBW	(%)	Controls	(%)
'Small' ($\leqslant$154 cm)	64	(43.0)	48	(32.2)
'Medium' (155–162 cm)	59	(39.6)	71	(47.7)
'Tall' ($\geqslant$163 cm)	26	(17.4)	30	(20.1)
Total	149	(100.0)	149	(100.0)

$\chi^2 = 3.68$, d.f. $= 2$, $p = 0.16$.

Table 3.8 Matching between LBW/control pairs for maternal height, using the 5 cm limit

Height difference	No. of pairs	(%)
LBW – C > 5 cm	5	(3.4)
LBW – C $\leqslant$ 5 cm	45	(30.2)
LBW = C	20	(13.4)
C – LBW $\leqslant$ 5 cm	51	(34.2)
C – LBW > 5 cm	28	(18.8)
Total	149	(100.0)

these cases having been selected on the basis of 'small', 'medium' or 'tall' (Table 3.8). The average height of the LBW mothers was 1.5 cm less than that of the controls—156.0 cm and 157.5 cm, respectively. This is reflected in the fact that 18.8 per cent of control mothers were more than 5 cm taller than the corresponding LBW mothers.

Accuracy of matching

When each of the matching criteria was considered separately, the distributions for the LBW and control groups were very similar, and no significant differences occurred when the chi-squared test was applied: similarly, a high percentage of pairs were accurately matched. Table 3.9 shows the proportions of LBW/control pairs accurately matched when all five criteria are considered together. 107 (71.8 per cent) of the pairs are matched with complete accuracy, and 144 (96.6 per cent) are matched on at least four of the five criteria.

Limitations of matching for environmental variables

In a study of child development it is desirable to control for environmental variables, which might otherwise obscure the findings. However, in a non-experimental setting, it is impossible to 'control' the environment with the

Table 3.9 Accuracy of matching

	No. of pairs	(%)
Matched on all 5 criteria	107	(71.8)
Matched on 4 criteria	37	(24.8)
Matched on 3 criteria	4	(2.7)
Matched on 2 criteria	1	(0.7)
Matched on 1 criterion	0	(0.0)
Total	149	(100.0)

degree of accuracy possible in a laboratory, where an experiment can be carried out in a closed system with every variable individually selected and monitored.

When the five variables selected as matching criteria in this study are examined, two issues arise: the fluctuations occurring beyond the control of the research worker and, related to this, the difficulty in defining categories of measurement. Only two of the five variables—sex of the child and height of the mother—can be guaranteed any permanency or ease of measurement over the duration of the study. The remaining three variables, smoking, social class, and child's ordinal number in the family, are all to some degree subject to change and so merit further consideration.

The child's ordinal number in the family can change when addition or removal of older siblings occurs, e.g. by remarriage of the child's parent to a new spouse with older children, by an older sibling being taken into care for a significant period of time, or by death.

The remaining two variables, in addition to being subject to change, also involve uncertainties in measurement. Maternal smoking behaviour was recorded at the antenatal booking visit in each case and this information was used as a basis for matching controls. However, some of the women stopped smoking during pregnancy and some increased the number of cigarettes smoked (see Chapter 4, page 79). Matching for smoking was not attempted on the basis of the number of cigarettes regularly smoked before pregnancy.

Social class, derived from the father's occupation, is the most complicated of the environmental variables used to match controls in this study: the following section and much of Chapters 4, 5 and 6 are concerned with its definition and meaning. In the context of this discussion, however, it is relevant to stress that attempts to measure social class by using the father's occupation can only give the crudest indication of the social environment in which these children were born and brought up, and this, like the other 'environmental' matching variables, can vary according to when it is recorded. Father's occupation was recorded twice for each of the families in the study, once at the mother's antenatal booking visit, when the information for matching controls was obtained, and once during the initial sociological interview after the delivery of the child. Eight of the fathers had moved to higher status occupations during this period and five had moved to lower status occupations. Of these, four had crossed the manual/non-manual boundary.

As the follow-up study progressed, the development of the North Sea oil industry brought new occupations to Aberdeen so that the list of occupational titles in 1979 would be different from that of 1970. There is, however, no reason to believe that these changes affected the sample and control groups differently.

SOCIO-ECONOMIC VARIABLES NOT SELECTED FOR MATCHING

Having selected the controls on the basis of father's occupation, a comparison of the study sample and controls on other social variables should demonstrate the degree to which similarity in the father's occupation indicates a broader similarity in socio-economic conditions. Other variables recorded at the time the study children were born were the mother's occupation before confinement, any previous mobility between occupations by either parent, the type of housing, the educational level achieved by the father (and, for primiparae, that of the mother*) and any further training completed by the father.

This comparison and the remainder of the sociological study are based on a reduced population of 286 out of the original 298 (149 LBW and 149 control). It was necessary to exclude 6 pairs because of incomplete sociological data.

MOTHER'S PREVIOUS OCCUPATION

For this variable, differences appeared between the two groups, the control mothers in general having higher status occupations than those in the LBW sample. Table 3.10 shows that 20.3 per cent of the controls compared with 7.7 per cent of the LBW mothers had a professional or technical occupation, and 23.1 per cent of the controls compared with 16.1 per cent of LBW mothers had clerical occupations. At the other end of the scale, 19.5 per cent of the LBW mothers were in semi-skilled occupations compared with 11.9 per cent of the controls, although the proportions in unskilled occupations were similar. Amongst the fishworkers, a group traditionally considered separately in Aberdeen due to their specific cultural, behavioural, and reproductive characteristics (Thompson 1977), 14.7 per cent of the LBW mothers are included compared with only 10.4 per cent of the controls. These distributions indicate an imbalance in social status between the study and control groups, in that many of the LBW mothers had not achieved the level of training and skill of their counterparts in the control group even though the occupational classes of their husbands were equivalent.

* The information was taken from the hospital record and is only recorded routinely for primiparae.

Table 3.10 Mother's previous occcupation

Occupational group	LBW	(%)	Controls	(%)
Professional/technical	11	(7.7)	29	(20.3)
Clerical	23	(16.1)	33	(23.1)
Distributive	26	(18.2)	21	(14.7)
Skilled manual	24	(16.8)	19	(13.3)
Semi-skilled manual	28	(19.5)	17	(11.9)
Unskilled	9	(6.3)	9	(6.3)
Fish worker	21	(14.7)	15	(10.4)
None	1	(0.7)	0	(0.0)
Total	143	(100.0)	143	(100.0)

$\chi^2 = 15.7$, d.f. $= 7$, $p = 0.0281$.

Occupational mobility

The women were asked to give the total work history of themselves and of their husbands. Although under detailed questioning they would be expected to give reasonably accurate accounts of their own jobs, some might not have been fully aware of their husband's history particularly if they had not known him for very long before marriage (e.g. when they were already pregnant). As Table 3.11 shows, the histories given were very similar in both LBW and control groups for the women and for their husbands when considered in terms of changes in status relative to the most recent job. The status of occupations was considered as either non-manual or manual and within these two broad groups mobility was assessed in terms of changes between the social classes, i.e. Social Class I, II, and IIIa in the non-manual group and IIIb, IV, and V in the manual group.

Equal numbers of LBW and control women had moved upwards (19), remained in the same group throughout (85), and moved downwards (39). Some of the downward mobility was associated with changes following marriage or pregnancy and more LBW women than controls had ended up in manual occupations when previously they had held non-manual jobs.

Consideration of husband's working histories shows that upward mobility had been similar for 29 LBW and 29 control husbands, but 33 LBW husbands had experienced downward mobility compared with 29 controls.

More fathers of control (65) than LBW (52) children had had one type of job only, which may indicate greater economic stability and security in the control families. This difference, however, did not reach statistical significance.

Type of housing

The housing arrangements of the LBW and control families were very similar

Table 3.11 Occupational mobility

Change in occupational status	Wives*				Husbands†			
	LBW	(%)	Controls	(%)	LBW	(%)	Controls	(%)
Upwards								
Non-manual, previously manual	4	(2.8)	6	(4.2)	9	(6.3)	9	(6.3)
Within non-manual or manual group	15	(10.5)	13	(9.1)	20	(14.0)	20	(14.0)
Unchanged								
One occupation only	70	(48.8)	72	(50.3)	52	(36.3)	65	(45.4)
Two or more occupations	15	(10.5)	13	(9.1)	29	(20.3)	20	(14.0)
Downwards								
Manual, previously non-manual	21	(14.7)	13	(9.1)	5	(3.5)	8	(5.6)
Within non-manual or manual group	18	(12.6)	26	(18.2)	28	(19.6)	21	(14.7)
Total	143	(100.0)	143	(100.0)	143	(100.0)	143	(100.0)

*$\chi^2 = 4.05$, d.f. $= 5$, $p = 0.5421$.
†$\chi^2 = 4.79$, d.f. $= 5$, $p = 0.4421$.

Table 3.12 House occupancy and sharing at birth of study child

House occupancy	LBW	(%)	Controls	(%)
Owner-occupier	35	(24.4)	42	(29.4)
Tenant unshared	69	(48.3)	64	(44.7)
Tenant/sub-let shared with others	39	(27.3)	37	(25.9)
Total	143	(100.0)	143	(100.0)

$\chi^2 = 0.88$, d.f. $= 2, p = 0.6450$.

(Table 3.12). Nearly half in each group were renting unshared council or private housing, but slightly more of the controls were owner-occupiers (24.2 per cent LBW, 29.4 per cent control). The remainder were sharing accommodation, usually with relatives.

Education and further training

Just over 80 per cent of both LBW and control fathers had left school at the minimum age (Table 3.13). Of those who received further training at a higher educational establishment (9.1 per cent LBW, 13.3 per cent control), significantly more control fathers attended for technical training (Table 3.14) and they were also more likely to have undertaken apprenticeships or vocational courses (Table 3.15).

Information available on primiparous women only (Table 3.16) shows that more control than LBW mothers had received vocational training (19.2 per cent LBW, 27.4 per cent control) but a similar proportion in each group had attended a university, teacher training college or equivalent.

Table 3.13 Father's school leaving age

School leaving age	LBW	(%)	Controls	(%)
Minimum school leaving age	116	(81.1)	116	(81.1)
16 years before 'O' grades	7	(4.9)	7	(4.9)
At 16/17 years after 'O' grades	7	(4.9)	4	(2.8)
After 17 years	9	(6.3)	15	(10.5)
Not stated	4	(2.8)	1	(0.7)
Total	143	(100.0)	143	(100.0)

$\chi^2 = 4.12$, d.f. $= 4, p = 0.3902$.

Table 3.14 Father's further education

Type of further education	LBW	(%)	Controls	(%)
None	127	(88.8)	124	(86.7)
Commercial college	3	(2.1)	1	(0.7)
Further education college (e.g. technical college)	2	(1.4)	9	(6.3)
University	8	(5.6)	9	(6.3)
Not stated	3	(2.1)	0	(0.0)
Total	143	(100.0)	143	(100.0)

$\chi^2 = 8.55$, d.f. $= 4$, $p = 0.0734$.

Table 3.15 Father's further training

Type of training	LBW	(%)	Controls	(%)
Armed forces	2	(1.4)	5	(3.5)
Apprenticeship	18	(12.6)	31	(21.7)
Other (day release, trade school, night school, in-service)	22	(15.4)	28	(19.6)
None/not continued	98	(68.5)	78	(54.5)
Not stated	3	(2.1)	1	(0.7)
Total	143	(100.0)	143	(100.0)

$\chi^2 = 8.73$, d.f. $= 4$, $p = 0.0683$.

Table 3.16 Mother's education (primiparae only)

Level of education	LBW	(%)	Controls	(%)
Minimum	51	(69.9)	44	(60.3)
Sixth form and further education (technical, vocational courses)	14	(19.2)	20	(27.4)
Higher education (colleges, university)	6	(8.2)	6	(8.2)
Not stated	2	(2.7)	3	(4.1)
Total	73	(100.0)	73	(100.0)

$\chi^2 = 1.77$, d.f. $= 3$, $p = 0.6205$.

Summary on socio-economic status

Of the variables recorded which indicate socio-economic status, the most noticeable differences between the LBW and control groups were in the excess of higher status occupations held by the control mothers, and the greater number of control fathers who had had some form of further education or training. Whilst mother's previous occupation was the only variable where the difference was statistically significant at a probability level of less than 5 per cent using the chi-squared test, the controls had a slight advantage over the LBW group for all the other variables, including job stability. The net effect of this imbalance yields a control group who are on average of a higher socio-economic status than their LBW counterparts.

COMPARISON OF THE LBW SAMPLE WITH THE POPULATION OF ORIGIN

Between July 1969 and June 1970, 177 singletons weighing 2500g or less and surviving at least 28 days were born in Aberdeen Maternity Hospital to women resident in Aberdeen City or suburbs. These 177 accounted for 6.2 per cent of the total comparable births in that year. Table 3.17 compares the characteristics of the LBW sample (145 babies) with the total LBW population which includes the 21 eligible babies who for various reasons were not recruited into the study and 11 babies known to be illegitimate (see Table 3.2).

The LBW sample comprised 82 per cent of the total LBW population and was not significantly different on any of the following criteria (which include four of the five criteria used in matching): social class, height, smoking, sex of infant, pregnancy number and parity (instead of ordinal position which was only available for the study population), maternal and paternal ages, and the mother's pre-marital occupation.

The controls were of course matched to the LBW population on the first four criteria listed in Table 3.17 which compares the total 149 controls with the total population of heavier babies for the 18-month period. Compared with all babies over 2500g, the controls were significantly different in all characteristics except for mother's age and occupation and baby's sex.

In summary, comparison of the LBW sample with the population of origin demonstrates that most of its characteristics are similar to those of the entire cohort. The controls acount for 3.6 per cent of the population from which they were taken and are clearly not a cross-section.

Finally, about 70 per cent of LBW babies weighed 2001−2500 g at birth and only 1 per cent weighed 1000 g or less. The birth weight of over one-quarter of the controls was 2501 g−3000 g and 42 per cent weighed 3000−3500 g. Thus, as Table 3.18 shows the distributions of birth weight in the two groups compared

Table 3.17 Comparison of LBW and control groups with their populations of origin

	Surviving singletons ≤2500 g July 1969–June 1970		Surviving singletons >2500 g July 1969–Dec 1970	
	LBW sample $N = 145$	Total ≤2500 g $N = 177$	Controls for LBW sample $N = 149$	Total >2500 g $N = 4144$
Social class				
% S.C. I and II	15.2	18.1*	16.8	21.5*
% S.C. IV and V	42.8	38.6*	38.9	24.5*
Maternal height				
% 'small' (≤154 cm)	43.4	41.8	32.2	21.0
% 'tall' (≥163 cm)	16.6	18.1	20.1	31.8
Maternal smoking				
% smokers	65.5	64.4	61.7	41.2
Sex of infant				
% male	49.7	44.6	49.7	51.7
Pregnancy no.				
% 1st	37.2	40.7	47.0	38.2
% 5+	10.3	10.2	6.7	4.9
Parity				
% para 0	49.0	51.4	51.0	42.5
% para 4+	4.1	4.0	4.7	2.4
Age of mother				
% <20	23.4	22.0	13.4	11.8
% 35+	11.7	10.7	3.4	5.5
Age of father				
% <20	9.7	8.4*	7.4	4.3*
% 35+	18.6	18.7*	5.4	10.8*
Mother's occupation†				
% Prof/tech	7.6	9.0	14.1	12.1
% Unskilled	7.6	6.8	2.0	3.5
% Fishworkers	12.4	11.9	8.7	5.8

* Per cent of total after excluding illegitimate infants.
† Mother's pre-marital occupation.

with their populations of origin are very similar and any differences are not statistically significant.

COMMENT

The justification for conducting a matched control study was the need to disentangle the specific influence of birth weight from that of environmental ex-

Table 3.18 Comparison of birth weight in LBW and control groups with those in the relevant cohorts of singleton deliveries

Sample period	Birth weight g	Sample %	Total births %
LBW	1000 or less	1.4	1.1
July 1969–June 1970	1001–1500	7.6	7.3
	1501–2000	22.1	19.8
	2001–2500	68.9	71.8
	Total	100	100
		(145)	(177)
Control	2501–3000	26.8	22.6
July 1969–December 1970	3001–3500	42.3	43.8
	3501–4000	27.5	26.9
	4001–4500	2.7	5.8
	4501 and over	0.7	0.9
	Total	100	100
		(149)*	(4144)

( ) Numbers.
* Includes the controls of additional 4 LBW cases born July–December 1970 who weighed 1840 g, 2330 g, 2430 g, 2482 g.

perience on later development and intellectual functioning. Thus close matching of variables related both sociologically and medically to the aetiology and outcome of low weight at birth was necessary in selecting a control group. Of the five variables used, perfect matching was only achieved for sex of the baby.

If it were possible to match perfectly for the social environment, subsequent differences in the intellectual and social development of LBW and control children could more plausibly be attributed to the major respect in which they differed, namely, birth weight; this, in turn, would facilitate the search for physiological and neurological differentiation factors at birth and in the neonatal period. Social class, closely correlated on the one hand with the incidence of LBW and on the other with indicators of child development, is obviously a key factor but it is a very crude measure of social environment and it was expected that three other socially related variables—family size, maternal smoking, and maternal height—would provide some measure of refinement.

In practice, it was not possible to obtain complete matching on these four variables although they were only broadly defined. The fact that, even so, complete matching could not be achieved for 149 index infants from a population of 3876 is an indication of the distinctive distribution of LBW. The two variables which presented most difficulty were maternal height and social class, particularly the combination of short stature and higher social class.

It was realized that the use of gross indicators at birth could predict the present and future environment of the child only in the most general way. Indeed, study of other socio-economic indicators immediately revealed an advantage to the control group, particularly with respect to the father's further training and the mother's pre-marital occupation, the latter being a variable which reflects the level of skill achieved by the mother and, jointly with paternal occupation, the social environment of the family. Since the family environment is so influential in child development, it clearly is of importance to investigate those other aspects of lifestyle which may differ between the study and control groups and may be influential in the future development of the child, but which are not controlled by crude matching for social class. Thus in Chapter 4 we discuss the contributions of certain environmental factors, parental relationships, and maternal aspirations, expectations, and behaviour to the mosaics which represent the varied patterns of family life.

Chapter 4

The Sociological Study: Differences Relevant to the Childhood Environment

M. RUSSELL, R. CARR-HILL AND R. ILLSLEY

INTRODUCTION

The question underlying the analyses in this chapter and in Chapter 9 is whether the observed lower performance of LBW children (compared to that of controls) on measures of outcome at 10 years can be attributed to environmental differences between LBW and control groups.

Most previous studies have adopted some form of categorization by social class. These measures have invariably shown a strong correlation with subsequent social, intellectual, and physical development. The precise meaning of social class and the mechanisms by which class is translated into degrees of performance will vary with the measures of outcome employed, e.g. in relation to physical development, class may signify nutrition and incidence of infection, whereas in relation to intellectual performance it may mean intellectual stimulation and educational training. Because of its pervasive nature and its value as a proxy indicator for many types of environmental experience, social class has assumed central importance in studies of birth weight and development.

At first sight the question may seem otiose, since the reason for studying matched pairs was precisely to control for environmental differences. Unfortunately, it is rarely possible in a sociological study to control as definitely as is sometimes possible in other fields of enquiry. Thus, although our examination of the accuracy of the matching in Chapter 3 demonstrated a high level of agreement, with 97 per cent of the pairs matched on at least four of the specified variables, it also revealed three inadequacies.

1. It had been necessary to relax the initial stringency of the matching criteria by adopting wider and therefore more heterogeneous groups for both social class and height. While this produced a formal match, it was nevertheless possible for LBW and control babies to differ by being drawn from different parts of the wider categories, e.g. for a Class III non-manual LBW baby to be paired with a Class I control.
2. The general tendency, within these broad categories, was for the LBW group to rank lower than the controls in class-related variables. Differences in the ordinal position in the family and in the husband's occupation were negligible but differences in maternal height were rather more substantial. This small but general tendency affecting three of the five criteria could result in controls having some advantage over the LBW group in the quality of the postnatal family environment.
3. Comparison of several non-matching variables indicative of the socioeconomic and educational level of the parents confirmed a residual difference between the LBW and control groups. If such factors as the mother's occupation and the husband's education exert a direct or indirect influence upon the postnatal environment (and there is good general evidence to this effect) we might expect the controls to perform better than LBW children on later measures of development for reasons not causally related to birth weight.

On these grounds alone it is important to study the characteristics of families as recorded in the postnatal sociological interview in some detail. But even if the match had been perfect (in terms of direct indicators of socio-economic status) there would have been another more general reason, viz. the variables used for matching, and the other occupational and educational variables compared in Chapter 3, refer to characteristics of the parents and the family before the birth of the index child: they have no direct implications for child-rearing practices and they are only crude indicators of social position and social behaviour. We know from other studies that occupational classes are extremely heterogeneous and that parents in, for example, Classes IV and V frequently provide more favourable child-rearing environments than a proportion of those in nominally more advantaged classes (Illsley, 1980). It is therefore of considerable importance to investigate those areas of the socio-cultural environment of the family which have been found in previous studies to affect the social and intellectual development of children.

The data collected at the postnatal interview are not necessarily the best possible for discriminating between child-rearing environments, as they are focused on the *intentions about* and *cultural factors related to* child-rearing rather than on *observed differences* in childhood experiences between birth and 10 years. However, given that all the other variables available for analysing the differences in outcome are general, medical or structural, they are likely to improve the prediction of outcome at 10 years.

The purpose of this chapter is to draw out from the questionnaire variables which reflect the environmental differences between LBW and control groups and which are likely to affect outcome at 10 years. These variables will then be included in the analyses in Chapter 9.

ANALYSING THE QUESTIONNAIRE DATA

A considerable number of questions were asked of the mothers (the complete questionnaire is available from the authors). The intention of these questions was to elicit information about five areas of the socio-cultural environment and the child-rearing intentions of the family. These were:

1. The socio-cultural background and the lifestyle of the family.
2. The aspirations and expectations of the mother for her child's development.
3. The mother's attitude to aspects of behaviour training.
4. The relationship between husband and wife in regard to child-rearing practices.
5. The amount of role rehearsal and planning for motherhood.

The kinds of questions asked in each block will be detailed more fully as we consider each section in turn.

There are two additional sources of data. The first is provided by subjective judgments made by the two interviewers. These relate to the mother's range of vocabulary, the fluency of her expression, and the organization and consistency of her thoughts revealed by her responses during the interview. The second is provided by the mother's responses to questions about intentions with regard to family planning.

As we have said, the ultimate purpose of the analyses in this chapter is to select variables from each section for use in regression analyses between potentially influential background factors and outcome measures obtained in psychological and medical examination of the children at 10 years. The distribution of answers to many specific questions did not vary between LBW and control groups and these will be omitted from the final regression analyses in Chapter 9. No tabulations are presented for these variables in this chapter although complete data are available from the authors.

However, there are too many variables which apparently discriminate between LBW and control groups for all of them to be included in the final analysis in Chapter 9, and we therefore need strategies for reducing the number to be considered. In the first place, intercorrelation of background variables suggested that discrimination obtained between LBW and control groups on some questions derived from their partial association with other and more powerful variables, and in these instances we have selected the latter for inclusion in the regression analyses in Chapter 9. In the second place, there are logical affinities between the questions asked in each of the sections and the observed intercorrelations of the answers to those questions.

Moreover, the subsequent analysis will relate *outcomes* at age 10 (Chapters 7 and 8) to variables presented in Chapters 4 and 5 measured at birth. While there may be some justification for linking, for example, neonatal problems to these outcomes, no similar 'causal' chain could be proposed linking the individual item responses to a sociological questionnaire completed postnatally to outcomes at age 10. We believe, however, that the individual item responses tap dimensions of child-rearing practices and socio-cultural environment which we suggest may have a valid relationship. Therefore, we have combined the responses to these separate questions—in relatively obvious ways—to form composite indices.

We have rejected 'automatic' data reduction techniques such as factor analyses, for two reasons. First, with such a small number of cases we want to retain control over the interpretation of our variables. Second, although there are logical affinities between the questions, they do not systematically overlap: for example, a couple's style of weekday evening activity is likely to be related to their weekend activity but these are partial measures of a larger whole rather than differently slanted measures of the same phenomenon.

We have proceeded as follows in each of the areas in turn: first, the individual items are analysed to see where the differences appear between LBW and control families; then the pattern of intercorrelations between the ranked variables within that area is examined to see which of the several dimensions included is most central to the area; and, finally, an index is constructed by adding together the ranked scores of those variables which also seem to reflect the same or a closely associated dimension within that area. Precise details of the rankings used and the construction of the indices are available in a Technical Appendix from the authors.

The amount of information which could be presented in this chapter is considerable and it seems unjustified to burden the reader with the detailed analysis. Accordingly, in general, we have presented only two tables for each section: one illustrative tabulation showing the variable in that group which most discriminates between LBW and control groups and a second table showing the relationship between the composite index and parents' age, parity, and social class. The correlation matrices of intercorrelations between the variables in each block and socio-economic status are given in the Appendix (Table 4.23, page 88). Other tables are obtainable from the authors.

The final output of this chapter will be a group of seven indices—two for socio-cultural environment and one each for the three child-rearing areas, the mother's preparation for motherhood, and the interviewers' assessment of the family, respectively. Finally, comment only is made on the families' intentions in regard to future fertility. We shall illustrate the importance of the indices by discussing their relationship with the five matching variables.

Socio-cultural background and lifestyle of the parents

Questions in this section of the interview related to:

The mother's pre-marital occupation
The mother's and father's main earlier occupations
School leaving age of fathers
School leaving age of mothers (primiparae only)
Further education and training of fathers
Further education and training of mothers (primiparae only)
Housing arrangements (owner-occupier, tenant, shared/unshared)
Parental ages
Duration of marriage
Working hours of fathers
Place of birth and upbringing of parents (Aberdeen; north-east Scotland; remainder of Scotland; elsewhere)
Recreational activities: (a) frequency of outings of mother and father together before pregnancy; (b) company on outings of couple—alone, with friends, with relatives, mixed; (c) indoor activities; (d) weekend activities

In Chapter 3 we reported a much heavier concentration of higher status occupations in the mothers of the control group and a tendency for both mothers and fathers of the control children to have received further education beyond the minimum school leaving age. There was no difference in housing arrangements. Additional information showed that more of the LBW group became unemployed between their first visit to the antenatal clinic and the postnatal interview and there was a tendency for more control fathers to work overtime or to be employed on shift work. In general, therefore, although not all these differences are significant, there is a clear indication from the occupational and educational histories that the control group has a higher socio-economic status.

This conclusion is supported by the further finding that control mothers were significantly less local in origin. Previous Aberdeen studies have shown (Illsley *et al.*, 1963) that migrants into Aberdeen are more likely to be drawn from higher socio-economic groups, to be taller and to have a healthier record in terms of obstetric mortality and morbidity. Nevertheless, the great majority of both parents in both groups were local in origin (nearly 80 per cent of controls and LBW fathers: 86 per cent of LBW mothers) and one or both of the spouses had relatives in the area. In both groups approximately one-fifth of the families were living with relatives and of the remainder the majority saw one or more relatives at least twice a week.

The most striking differences, however, are between the ages of parents of LBW and control children, for while the *average* ages of mothers and fathers do not differ significantly as between LBW and controls the *distributions* are very different (Table 4.1). Notwithstanding the fact that the proportion of control mothers aged under 25 was significantly higher than that for the total population of mothers, the LBW group contained an excess of mothers both in their teens (23 per cent LBW, 13 per cent control) and aged 35 or over (10 per cent LBW, 2 per cent control). This pattern also appears when primiparae and multiparae are considered separately, being particularly significant for primiparae ($p < 0.02$).

Table 4.1   Percentage of mothers and fathers in each age group at the childs birth (143 unmatched pairs)

Age (years)	Mothers		Fathers	
	LBW	Control	LBW	Control
−19	23.1	13.3	9.8	7.0
19−24	32.8	49.6	33.5	35.6
25−29	24.5	25.9	25.9	37.1
30−34	9.8	9.1	12.6	14.7
35−39	9.1	2.1	10.5	4.9
40+	0.7	—	6.3	—
not stated	—	—	1.4	0.7
Significance of χ^2, p	0.007		0.013	

The aetiology of low birth weight is likely to be very different as between the very young and the oldest mothers. Thus, the low birth weight of the baby of an older mother is likely to be due, at least in part, to ageing and atrophy of maternal tissues which are also conducive of other abnormalities in the baby. Although women age differently there is no particular reason to suppose that these differences would be associated with intentions about child-rearing practices and the socio-cultural environment at the time of birth of a particular child.

On the other hand, low birth weight in babies of young mothers (especially primiparae) is likely to be due to physiological immaturity, which, in turn, may be due to deprivation during childhood and adolescence. In this case, it is reasonable to suppose that differences in the level of deprivation would be indicated by differences in intentions about child-rearing practices and in the socio-cultural environment.

Inasmuch as low birth weight can be attributed to socio-cultural disadvantage which may not be reflected by social class (which was used as a matching variable), one would expect the effect to be more noticeable with the younger mothers. This possibility is so crucial for the subsequent interpretations that the mother's age has been retained as a classification variable throughout this chapter, as if it were a matching variable.

We are left with a collection of variables which reflect the social and cultural background of the parents and which discriminate between the LBW and control groups taken as a whole, although not always significantly. In order to derive a meaningful measure of the differences between the LBW and control groups we have chosen one variable from each of the four areas, viz. the mother's working life, the living conditions at home, the father's educational attainment and the geographical mobility of the mother.

A composite index has been constructed by adding together the ranked scores obtained in response to the following questions:

Mother's last occupation ranked according to status
House occupancy ranked according to security of tenure
Husband's further training present or absent
Mother's place of upbringing ranked according to distance from Aberdeen

This index of *mobility and professional status* can range in value from 3 to 18. Table 4.2 shows the distribution between LBW and controls and in the total study population. For the purposes of further analysis these values have been bracketed as follows: 8 or less, signifying low mobility and professional status; between 9 and 12, signifying average status; and 13 and over, signifying high mobility and professional status. With this grouping there is a significant difference between LBW and controls, $\chi^2 = 7.29$, $p = <0.03$.

Table 4.2   Index of mobility and professional status: distribution in LBW and control groups.

	3−6	7−8	9−10	11−12	13−14	15−16	Total
LBW	9	44	36	19	26	9	143
Controls	12	21	40	21	29	20	143
	21	65	76	40	55	29	286

When the index is broken down according to mother's age and parity and separately according to husband's social class (see Table 4.3 (a), (b)) we find that there are significant differences amongst young primiparous mothers and amongst mothers married to husbands in Social Class IIIb. These differences are substantial: for example, among young primiparous mothers nearly half the LBW mothers score 8 or less while nearly three-quarters of the control mothers score 9 or more. Thus, even within tightly circumscribed groups, there are differences between the LBW and control families in their mobility and professional status. The environment of the control child is likely to be more rich and varied.

Table 4.3   Index of mobility and professional status (a) according to mother's age and parity and (b) separately according to social class

(a)

| | Mother's age | | | | | | | | |
| | Under 25 | | | | 25–49 | | | |
	8 and under	Index 9–12	13 and more	Total	8 and under	Index 9–12	13 and more	Total
Primiparae								
LBW	22	22	9	53	3	4	13	20
Controls	16	23	23	62	1	3	7	11
Total	38	45	32	115	4	7	20	31
Multiparae								
LBW	15	10	2	27	13	19	11	43
Controls	9	16	3	28	7	19	16	42
Total	24	26	5	55	20	38	27	85

(b)

| | Social Class | | | | | | | | | | | |
| | I–IIIa | | | | IIIb | | | | IV–V | | | |
	8 and under	Index 9–12	13 and more	Total	8 and under	Index 9–12	13 and more	Total	8 and under	Index 9–12	13 and more	Total
LBW	1	12	20	33	16	25	10	51	36	18	5	59
Controls	2	5	26	33	6	33	15	54	25	23	8	56
Total	3	17	46	66	22	58	25	105	61	41	13	115

Table 4.4 Percentage in groups according to number of evening and weekend activities (143 matched pairs)

No. of activities		LBW	Control	p
Evening*				
At home	0	11.2	9.1	
	1	41.3	26.5	0.015
	2	47.5	64.4	
Weekend				
	1	35.0	19.6	0.005
	2+	65.0	80.4	

* TV and reading excluded.

The questions on recreational activity were designed to reveal the width of interests of activities of the parents individually and as couples and also to tap the quality of the activity particularly as regards its intellectual and cultural content. There were significant differences between LBW and control groups in some of the questions on recreational activities, the most striking occurring in the number of evening and weekend activities (see Table 4.4) and the type of weekend activity. The pattern of intercorrelations (see Appendix) suggests that the key organizing concept is the level of activity/passivity involved in the recreation rather than the frequency or amount of time spent. The interpretation is reinforced by the fact that the statistically significant intercorrelations are concentrated on the first-named weekend recreation.

We suggest, therefore, that a composite index reflecting the differences in socio-cultural environment can be constructed by adding together the ranked scores from the mother's responses to questions on evening and weekend activities, as follows:

They usually go out in the evening with other people
Their first mentioned weekend activity is not TV
They mention more than one weekend activity
They mention more than one evening activity in addition to TV and reading

This index of *recreational activity* can have values between 4 and 16. They are distributed between the LBW and controls as in Table 4.5. For the sake of fur-

Table 4.5 Index of recreational activity: distribution in LBW and control groups.

	8.5 and under	9–10	10.5–11	11.5–12	12.5	13 and over	Total
LBW	22	36	29	29	18	9	143
Controls	9	25	30	25	28	26	143
Total	31	61	59	54	46	35	286

Table 4.6   Index of recreational activity (a) by mother's age and parity and (b) separately by social class

(a)

	Mother's age							
	Under 25				25 and over			
	10 and under	Index 10.5–12	over 12	Total	10 and under	Index 10.5–12	over 12	Total
Primiparae								
LBW	17	27	9	53	2	9	9	20
Controls	11	21	30	62	1	3	7	11
Total	28	48	39	115	3	12	16	31
Multiparae								
LBW	17	8	2	27	22	14	7	43
Controls	7	15	6	28	15	16	11	42
Total	24	23	8	55	37	30	18	85

(b)

	Social Class											
	I–IIIa				IIIb				IV–V			
	10 and under	Index 10.5–12	over 12	Total	10 and under	Index 10.5–12	over 12	Total	10 and under	Index 10.5–12	over 12	Total
LBW	6	15	12	33	21	20	10	51	31	23	5	59
Controls	2	8	23	33	15	25	14	54	17	22	17	56
Total	8	23	35	66	36	45	24	105	48	45	22	115

ther analysis the index has been grouped into three categories: 10 or less, more than 10 and up to 12, more than 12. With this concatenation, the differences between LBW and controls are highly significant ($\chi^2 = 15.3$, $p < 0.01$). It is clear that the procedure of matching on the five specified variables did not eliminate overall differences between LBW and control groups in terms of their propensity to engage in what are considered to be culturally 'active' as against 'inactive' pursuits.

The overall differences observed do not, however, necessarily imply that there are such cultural differences within particular socially defined sub-groups. The data in Table 4.6 give the breakdown of the index according to the mother's age and parity and separately according to the husband's social class. The χ^2 statistics for this and similar tables are presented together in Table 4.7. The data suggest that while there are significant differences for younger mothers irrespective of parity, the differences disappear with older mothers. Moreover, there are significant differences within Social Classes I–IIIa and IV–V. Clearly, neither the matching for parity nor the matching by social class has eliminated differences between LBW and controls in terms of the likelihood that they pursue active cultural pursuits. And these differences are substantial: thus over four-fifths of the control mothers among the young primiparae score over 10 while nearly one-third of the LBW mothers score 10 or less. Similarly, while over two-thirds of controls among social classes I–IIIa score more than 12, nearly two-thirds of the LBW mothers score 12 or less.

Thus LBW babies, irrespective of social class and particularly if born to young mothers, may from the beginning suffer disadvantages due to the limited social experience and restricted contacts and activities of their parents.

Expectations of influencing the child's physical and intellectual development, and attitudes to education

Differences in attitudes and expectations between middle and lower social class groups have been observed in several comparative studies. The culture of poverty theorists (Spinley, 1953; Lewis, 1966) propose that the lowest classes (i.e. the very poor who possess little skill or property and experience intermittent or long-term unemployment) hold a separate system of values and norms which guide and help to explain their behaviour. On an individual level, characteristics of this sub-group include feelings of powerlessness and fatalism, a present-time rather than future orientation, and a lack of belief in being able to control major life events. A lack of integration or participation with other social strata helps to maintain the existence of this sub-culture. The situational model (Davis 1946) explains differences in lower working class behaviour in terms of response to a lack of economic resources, educational and occupational opportunity, social status, and political power. Although this model acknowledges that different norms and values may result from economic and

Table 4.7 Values of chi-squared and their associated significance levels for the differences observed between LBW and control families in respect of the seven indices when analysed according to mother's age and parity and separately according to father's social class

| | | | Indices | | | | |
	I Socio-cultural environment (a)	I Socio-cultural environment (b)	2 Expectations to influence child	3 Behaviour training	4 Husband's participation	5 Preparation for motherhood	6 Interviewer's assessment
Primiparae							
Mother's age							
under 25 χ^2	6.42	12.72	8.63	7.78	3.55	6.32	5.54
p	0.04*	0.002†	0.013*	0.021*	0.17	0.043*	0.063
25 and over χ^2	0.36	1.06	0.71	9.52	1.94	1.74	0.57
p	0.84	0.59	0.70	0.009†	0.38	0.42	0.75
Multiparae							
Mother's age							
under 25 χ^2	3.07	8.28	0.046	2.06	6.16	5.54	3.80
p	0.22	0.016*	0.79	0.36	0.046*	0.065	0.15
25 and over χ^2	2.71	2.34	2.23	8.44	1.04	5.08	10.14
p	0.26	0.31	0.33	0.015*	0.59	0.079	0.006†
Social Class							
I–IIIa χ^2	4.00	7.89	8.16	6.47	0.089	0.37	2.25
p	0.14	0.023*	0.017*	0.039*	0.96	0.83	0.32
IIIb χ^2	6.57	2.14	4.88	5.15	4.14	4.51	7.97
p	0.038*	0.34	0.087	0.076	0.13	0.11	0.019*
IV–V χ^2	3.21	10.58	2.46	11.07	4.29	3.26	6.92
p	0.20	0.005†	0.292	0.004†	0.12	0.20	0.031*
All cases χ^2	7.29	15.34	6.19	20.25	6.65	4.84	13.83
p	0.026*	0.005†	0.045*	0.0005†	0.036*	0.089	0.001†

* Significant at 5% level.
† Significant at 1% level.

social deprivation, the situation itself rather than a cultural difference is held as the cause of differing behaviour patterns. Chamberlain (1976) also used this explanation in her study of high parity women.

The adaptational model combines elements of both cultural and situational explanations: it has been used by Kreisberg (1963) to explain differences between lower working class and middle class behaviour in voting, achievement of college education, and use of medical and dental care, and by Askham (1975) in her examination of lower working class fertility. Askham described four characteristics of lower working class members which may be viewed as culturally different from those of other social groups, and resulting, at least in part, from situational factors. These are: 1. an orientation towards the present rather than the future; 2. an attitude of fatalism and inability to control major life events; 3. an inability (or lack of belief in personal ability) to influence wider events, e.g. politically or within the community; and 4. an inability to improve material well-being and esteem.

For the purposes of the present study it is worth bearing in mind that, although any such cultural sub-group may be expected to occur only within the lowest social class (since the three models described above were based on studies of lower working class behaviour), it is possible that people with these orientations may be found in other social groups as well. Conversely, as Kreisberg (1963) points out, not all members of the lowest social class should be expected to display these sub-cultural characteristics.

The women in the Aberdeen LBW study were asked during the hospital interview about their beliefs in their abilities to influence their child's physical and intellectual development, to find out if they exhibited signs of the sub-cultural characteristics described above. Apart from theoretical considerations, any sub-group oriented to the present and with attitudes of fatalism and powerlessness in facing the future, will be an important group to study when the children are followed up in 10 years, since these children are the least likely to receive environmental stimulation during their development and, if they are of low birth weight, their progress may be doubly disadvantaged.

Other studies not concerned particularly with models for lower working class behaviour have also noted differences in expectations in lower social classes. For example, Kagan and Tulkin (1971) in their study of mother–infant interaction noted that working class mothers were less likely to regard themselves as able to influence their children's development, and that this group in fact stimulated their infants less than middle class mothers.

Several studies have considered attitudes to education and ambitions. For example, Wilmott and Young (1960) found that some working class parents in London were just as ambitious for their children to achieve grammar school places as were the middle class parents, and Klein (1965) in her extensive review of child-rearing in differing English cultures concluded that middle class parents were more concerned with educational performance and supervised both schoolwork and leisure time activities more closely than working class parents. This difference in the level of achievement motivation between different social classes is attributed by McClelland *et al.* (1953) to differential class emphasis on independence and achievement training, whereby middle class parents are more likely to stress self-reliance, autonomy, and achievement in problem-solving situations.

In summary, the characteristic attitudes and expectations found in *some* members of the lower social classes, which may be a consequence of differing situational factors, offer an explanation for differences between lower and middle class behaviour. For the present purposes it is suggested that certain of these sub-cultural characteristics constitute a more sensitive index of the social environment and therefore may be useful in discriminating between women within the same social class, in both the LBW and control groups.

In the interview, the mothers were asked whether they expected to have any influence on when the child would begin to crawl, walk or talk, how much they expected to help the child in schoolwork and whether they would teach the child to read before going to school.

The control mothers were consistently more positive in their expectations to

Table 4.8   Mother's expectation of influencing the child to talk, to read, and in school progress

	LBW %	Control %	p
To talk			
(143 matched pairs)			
Yes	79.0	85.3	
Uncertain	0.7	2.1	
No	12.6	5.6	0.18
No—will talk when ready	5.6	6.3	
No comment	2.1	0.7	
To read			
(104 matched pairs)			
Yes	47.1	37.6	
Only if child interested	5.8	16.3	0.02
Uncertain	12.5	21.1	
No	34.6	25.0	
In school progress			
(143 matched pairs)			
Yes	56.6	67.1	
Only if child interested	28.0	25.9	
Uncertain	2.8	3.5	0.05
No	11.2	3.5	
No comment	1.4	—	

influence their child to crawl, walk or talk than the LBW parents, although the differences were never significant. Significant differences did occur, however, in comparing the proportions who did *not* expect to influence their child in reading or in school progress (see Table 4.8).

The four types of maternal expectation to influence the child (to crawl, to walk, to talk, and to do well at school) all intercorrelate significantly. Belief in the effect of environmental influences (as opposed to heredity) on educational development correlates with the expectation to influence speech acquisition and school progress. The intention to teach the child to read correlates with none of these expectations and attitudes. It also differs in that it is negatively related to social class whereas the others are positively related. Inspection of the responses suggests that the upper social groups and the control mothers were more hesitant about teaching their children to read because of the possibility that their methods would later conflict with those of the school.

In view of these findings it seems appropriate to group the four intercorrelated variables relating to the expectation to influence the child's development into a composite index to reflect the mother's belief in her ability to control or influence the environment as opposed to hereditary or fatalistic views. Thus, a composite index has been constructed by adding together the ranked scores obtained from the mothers' responses to questions on their expectation to influence the child's development, as follows:

They expect to influence crawling
They expect to influence walking
They expect to influence talking
They expect to help the child at school
They think a child's progress is influenced by the environment, or by a mixture of heredity and environment

This index of *belief in ability to influence the environment* can range in value from 4 to 12. It is distributed among the LBW and controls as in Table 4.9. In order to construct detailed analysis the index has been grouped into three categories (7 or less, 8, 9 or more): with this grouping the differences between LBW and controls are significant ($\chi^2 = 6.19$, $p > 0.05$). Once again the conclusion must be that the overall differences between LBW and control groups have

Table 4.9 Index of belief in ability to influence the environment: distribution in LBW and control groups

	6 and under	7	8	9	10	11 or 12	Total
LBW	23	28	35	19	20	18	143
Controls	20	19	26	26	30	22	143
Total	43	47	61	45	50	40	286

Table 4.10   Index of belief in ability to influence the environment (a) by mother's age and parity and (b) separately by social class

(a)

	Mother's age							
	Under 25				25 and over			
		Index				Index		
	7 and under	8	9 and over	Total	7 and under	8	9 and over	Total
Primiparae								
LBW	25	8	20	53	4	4	12	20
Controls	14	9	39	62	3	1	7	11
Total	39	17	59	115	7	5	19	31
Multiparae								
LBW	8	10	9	27	14	13	15	42
Controls	9	8	11	28	13	8	21	42
Total	17	18	20	55	27	21	36	84

(b)

	Social Class											
	I–IIIa				IIIb				IV–V			
		Index				Index				Index		
	7 and under	8	9 and over	Total	7 and under	8	9 and over	Total	7 and under	8	9 and over	Total
LBW	7	10	16	33	18	16	17	51	26	9	24	59
Controls	2	4	27	33	19	8	27	54	18	14	24	56
Total	9	14	43	66	37	24	44	105	44	23	48	115

not been eliminated by matching on the five specified variables. The parents of LBW and control groups are different in respect of their expectation to influence their children's development in the basic skills.

However, we cannot take these overall differences as necessarily implying that such differences in child-rearing practices exist in particular social groups. Table 4.10 shows the breakdown of the index according to mother's age and parity and, separately, according to the husband's social class. The only significant differences are with young primiparous mothers and with mothers married to husbands of Social Class I, II, and IIIa (see Table 4.7) but it is important to notice that these differences are quite substantial. Thus, among young primiparous mothers over 60 per cent of LBW mothers score 8 or less, while over 60 per cent of control mothers score 9 or more: similarly, among mothers married to husbands in Social Classes I, III, and IIIa over half of the LBW mothers score 8 or less while over four-fifths of the control mothers score 9 or more.

Once again, therefore, and even within the upper social classes, the LBW mothers and especially young primiparae are more fatalistic and have less expectations of being able to influence the environment or help their child in reaching the milestones of development or in educational achievement. The stimulus of a creative environment therefore favours the control children.

Behaviour training

Many studies of child-rearing in recent years have demonstrated the variation between classes and cultures in child training behaviour (e.g. Davis and Havinghurst, 1946; Sears et al., 1957; Newson and Newson, 1963). Changes in class and cultural behaviour over time have made categorizations of class differences in approaches to child-rearing appear inconsistent or ambiguous. For example, Davis and Havinghurst (1946) in Chicago, in one of the first major studies of social class differences in child-rearing, concluded that middle class children were being reared more restrictively than working class children. They based this view on the more rigid feeding schedules, earlier weaning and toilet training, and earlier allocation of domestic responsibilities undertaken in middle class households, compared with the observed permissiveness over these issues in working class households. In addition, a higher reported frequency of masturbation and thumbsucking in middle class households was interpreted as indicating that the children were reacting to the frustration of their natural impulses by the imposition of these training practices.

In a later study of New England families Sears et al. (1957), using a slightly different interpretation of the observed behaviour of their middle and working class families, concluded that their middle class mothers were on the whole gentler and more permissive in many areas of child-rearing, especially over dependency behaviour by the child and sex exploration. They were less punitive in general and less likely to use physical punishment when disciplining their children. These authors noticed no differences between rigidity of feeding schedules and the ages at which weaning and toilet training were commenced, although they noted that working class mothers completed toilet training two and a half months earlier on average and were more likely to use scolding and 'shaming' for failure to achieve bladder control. By emphasizing class differences in behaviour training and by finding no differences in those areas which had led Davis and Havinghurst to their conclusions, they were able to suggest that working class mothers were more punitive and middle class mothers more permissive in their approach to childrearing. Kohn and Carroll (1960), in a classic article, showed that the differences between these studies were not necessarily contradictory in that each could have accurately portrayed behaviour at the time of the study itself.

In Nottingham, Newson and Newson (1963) were able to demonstrate social class differences in different areas of child-rearing. These indicated varying levels of permissiveness and punitiveness over different issues in differing social classes, revealing similarities to both sets of American data. For instance, as in Chicago, middle class women in Nottingham set higher goals in general for their children and started weaning and potty training earlier. In addition, middle class mothers tended to put their children to bed earlier and to refrain from using a bottle or dummy as a comforter if the child woke at night. However, middle class mothers were not portrayed as being overly 'strict' in this study. For instance, their babies were not left to cry any longer if they woke at night and, although these mothers were less permissive about continued sucking as evidenced by their reluctance to use bottles and dummies after starting to wean the child, their methods of discouraging the child were recorded as being 'gentle discouragement, distraction, and very gentle change'. Early weaning in itself was attributed partly to the greater preference for breast feeding among the middle class mothers, in whom drying-up of breast milk may have forced the issue sooner than if a bottle had been used. Working class women, however, were not always more permissive, for they tended to punish their children more often and to smack more freely for many offences, particularly failure to use the potty and genital play, than did middle class mothers. An additional observation in this study was the greater tendency towards inconsistency in behaviour amongst Social Class V mothers, some of whom would react to misbehaviour by first of all slapping the child and then offering a sweet or dummy to get over the slap, or by ignoring a certain type of misbehaviour on one occasion and punishing it on another. This type of inconsistency was proposed by these authors as a factor in the greater frequency of temper tantrums in this social class, which they attributed to frustration in the small child.

The picture emerging of British mothers in the 1960s is of middle class mothers who exert greater pressure on their children to achieve certain goals but who are selective about their use of punishment, and physical punishment in particular, espeically in areas such as toilet training and genital play where some psychological damage may be thought to follow. In the working class pattern, punishment features more strongly as a training method but certain restrictive middle class practices such as early bedtime and repression of sucking behaviour are not favoured. The questions posed in our sociological interview were designed to reveal these dimensions in behaviour training.

Class differences in child-rearing practice are not necessarily due to differences in ideology. For some parents a compromise has to be reached due to the constraints imposed by the social environment. This point has relevance to many areas of child-rearing: for example, the amount of husband participation in child-rearing is automatically limited by his working hours; the degree of permissiveness over toilet training may be strongly influenced by the availability of hot water for nappy washing. Housing conditions, too, will affect the freedom with which a mother can allow her child to play safely and the amount of noise a child can make without disturbing neighbours. Similarly, the length of time a baby can be left to cry will depend on whether the crying will waken other children asleep in the same room. Class differences in child-rearing may thus be the product of many influences, some rooted in class cultures, some due to changing fashions in child-rearing, and some due to material circumstances.

The connection between child-rearing practices and child development is at best rather tenuous and few studies have examined it systematically. The only sociological study which attempted to trace links between the mother's treatment of the child and his later behaviour was that of Sears et al. (1957) who noted the association of feeding problems, bed wetting, aggressive behaviour, and lowering of conscience development with maternal 'coldness' (defined as lack of affection, demonstrativeness, and response to the child's dependency behaviour, combined with very little reasoning in behaviour training and little praise for good behaviour). These authors also noted a failure in the effectiveness of severe punishment in changing the behaviour for which it was administered, e.g. mothers who punished their children severely for aggressive behaviour frequently ended up with more aggressive children than did those who only punished their children slightly for similar behaviour. The same was true of punishment of dependency behaviour and for failure to use the potty. However, it was pointed out that the punishment itself may not have been the sole cause of this effect, since the children in question may have had a higher rate of aggression/dependency/resistance to potty training initially.

Much work, particularly that of psychologists, has been less concerned with child-rearing practices than with the effect of mother–infant relationships and parental separation on the child's social and intellectual development. This research has shown that normal social development in young children is related to maternal sensitivity, acceptance, co-operation and accessibility, which foster a secure mother–infant attachment which the young child may use as a basis for exploring and learning about the wider environments (Ainsworth et al., 1974). The formation of an early stable mother–infant bond was regarded for many years as crucial to the normal social development of the child, and many adult disorders such as delinquency and psychopathy have been attributed to impairments in the capacity to form bonds of affection, often as a result of inadequate mother–infant bonding in infancy (Bowlby 1952; Ainsworth 1962). However, inadequate or disrupted bonding with the mother in infancy is only one of a group of adverse early life experiences, known collectively as 'maternal deprivation', which may impair normal social, emotional, and intellectual development. For instance, privation of perceptual and linguistic experience has been shown to contribute to developmental retardation and intellectual impairment. Delinquency may be a consequence of family discord and psychopathy a long-term consequence of failure to develop bonds in the first three years of life, while acute distress immediately following maternal separation may be due to a disruption of the bonding process (Rutter, 1972, 1979). Emotional disorders in children following parental separation have not been found to be related to the event of separation *per se*, but rather to any family distress or discord which may have precipitated the separation. Rutter (1971), for example, found no long-term ill effects in children separated from their parents for holidays or admission to hospital. There are of course many intervening variables such as the child's age and sex or the presence of other attachment figures, which may alter the child's response to deprivation, but a discussion of these would be inappropriately lengthy for present purposes.

Psychological studies have also demonstrated social class differences in parent–child interactions. Thus Kagan and Tulkin (1971) attributed higher verbal competence, sustained attention and inhibition in middle class two-year-olds to the higher level of stimulation and longer periods of vocalization by their mothers, when compared to a similar group of working class mothers and children. However, middle and working class mothers were not found to display any differences in the affective elements of mother–infant interaction, such as kissing and holding the baby. These differences in verbalization and stimulation may relate to the underlying class differences in maternal beliefs about influencing child development discussed in the previous section.

Questions in the sociological interview relevant to behaviour training covered three different areas:

1. *Infant care and routines*   What would you do if he/she wakes up during the night?
   (a) Nurse until settles down
   (b) Take into parents' bed
   (c) Leave to cry
   (d) Other.
   As regards feeding, what type of routine might you choose?
   (a) Demand
   (b) Fixed schedule
   (c) Other.

2. *Infant behaviour*   What would you do if he/she plays with his/her body much?
   (a) Scratches face/pulls hair
   (b) Sucks thumb
   (c) Sucks other objects
   (d) Plays with genitals.
3. *Child behaviour*   How do you think you might react to the following situations?
   (a) If your child was singing and you had a bad headache?
   (b) If your child insisted on dominating the conversation at the dinner table?
   (c) If your child was drawing on good writing paper?
   (d) If your child became friendly with a child whom you considered an undesirable friend?
   (e) When small children use naughty words—ignore, punish, laugh it off?

Mothers of LBW babies were significantly different from controls in their attitudes towards the baby crying at night if they were certain that nothing was wrong, a higher proportion being more likely to pick the baby up at once or to leave him to cry himself to sleep. The two groups did not differ, however, in their intentions to use a dummy or take the child into their own bed. Nor did they differ in preferences for flexible or formal daily routines. However, the difference between the two groups in their feeding routines was highly significant; LBW mothers in the immediate postnatal period were more conscious of the necessity to adapt their routines to the prior needs of a small infant (see Table 4.11).

Control mothers were significantly more permissive in their attitudes to thumb-sucking and to the sucking of other objects but there were no differences in relation to playing with the genitals. They were also more permissive in their attitudes towards the child using bad language but the two groups were similar in their responses to the other four aspects of child behaviour (see above).

Table 4.11   Reasons for choosing a particular feeding routine (143 matched pairs)

Reason	LBW %	Control %
Small baby needs regular feeds	2.8	0.7
Same as hospital/special nursery	9.8	2.1
Not waken baby to feed	34.2 } 51.0	49.6 } 60.1
Baby makes his own routine	16.8	10.5
Mother needs a routine	9.8	18.2
Did the same with previous child	2.8	5.6
Best for baby	7.7	4.9
No comment	11.9	7.0
Routine unknown	4.2	1.4

$\chi^2 = 24.66$, d.f. $= 8, p = 0.0018$.

The pattern of intercorrelations (see Appexdix page 88) shows that the responses towards the child crying at night, although differentiating between LBW and control groups, did not correlate significantly with the other aspects of infant and child behaviour in which the two groups differed. Similarly, although there were consistent correlations between the proposed reactions to infant sucking and genital behaviour they did not correlate significantly with the other aspects of behaviour training. Finally, the mother's reactions to different types of child behaviour were apparently all independent of one another. It seems clear that there are three 'types' of differences between the LBW and the control mothers in respect of their attitudes towards behaviour training.

Because of these, three separate indices have been constructed corresponding to the three components of behaviour training identified above. In fact, the only index which showed systematic differences between LBW and control mothers was that related to the expected reactions to 'naughty' child behaviour. The index was constructed by adding together the ranked scores obtained in response to questions on child behaviour ((a), (d), and (e) in area 3. Child Behaviour page 71).

This index of *behaviour training* (degree of intervention and 'strictness') ranges in value between 3 and 16. It is distributed in the study population and separately among the LBW parents and the control group of parents as shown in Table 4.12. While the values of the index are fairly evenly distributed amongst the population, there are sharp differences between LBW and controls. Thus, when we group the index in three categories—under 6, 6 and under 8, 8 and over—we obtain a χ^2 of 20.25 ($p < 0.001$) which is highly significant. Once again, the conclusion is that there are overall differences between the LBW and control group, this time in respect of their attitudes towards behaviour training.

The breakdown according to mother's age and parity and husband's social class is given in Table 4.13. There are significant differences for young primiparous mothers and older multiparous mothers and a highly significant difference is obtained for older primiparous mothers (see Table 4.7). Note, however, that the differences among older primiparous mothers are not consistent between the three categories of the index. There is also a significant difference for mothers married to husbands in Social Classes I, II or IIIa and a highly significant difference for mothers married to husbands in Social Classes

Table 4.12   Index of behaviour training: distribution in LBW and control groups

	4 and under	4.5–5.5	6–6.5	7–7.5	8–9.5	10 and over	Total
LBW	13	23	19	21	43	24	143
Controls	23	20	40	28	22	10	143
Total	36	43	59	49	65	34	286

Table 4.13 Index of behaviour training (a) by mother's age and parity and (b) separately by social class

(a)

	Mother's age							
	Under 25				25 and over			
	Index				Index			
	5.5 and under	6–7.5	8 and over	Total	5.5 and under	6–7.5	8 and over	Total
Primiparae								
LBW	10	15	28	53	9	4	7	20
Controls	17	28	17	62	3	8	0	11
Total	27	43	45	115	12	12	7	31
Multiparae								
LBW	8	8	11	27	9	13	21	43
Controls	8	13	7	28	15	19	8	42
Total	16	21	18	55	24	32	29	85

(b)

	Social Class											
	III–IIIa				IIIb				IV–V			
	Index				Index				Index			
	5.5 and under	6–7.5	8 and over	Total	5.5 and under	6–7.5	8 and over	Total	5.5 and under	6–7.5	8 and over	Total
Primiparae												
LBW	9	11	13	33	18	15	18	51	9	14	36	59
Controls	14	15	4	33	16	27	11	54	13	26	17	56
Total	23	26	17	66	34	42	29	105	22	40	53	115

IV and V. Moreover, some of these differences are substantial: thus among young primiparous mothers over half of the LBW mothers score 8 or more while nearly three-quarters of the control mothers score less than 8; similarly, amongst mothers married to husbands in social classes IV or V, over 60 per cent of LBW mothers score 8 or more while nearly 70 per cent of control mothers score less than 8.

The more permissive, less punitive attitude of control mothers, especially of older women having their first baby, and the social class differences suggest the influence of child-rearing theories, e.g. Spock (1957).

The role of the husband

At the time these interviews were conducted very little was known about the effect the father had on his child's emotional, behavioural, and intellectual development. His role in the early attachment behaviour of the infant was thought to be negligible or at best much inferior to the mother–infant relationship, which was assumed by the theorists of the day to be of paramount importance (Freud, 1940; Parsons, 1958; Bowlby, 1969). The differences between the models proposed by these theorists lay only in the nature of the advantage to the mother and infant of promoting and reinforcing the bond, and not in the initial assumption of its primary importance in the infant's life.

Essentially, this assumption was based on the rather loose argument that because the mother spends more time than anyone else with the infant, she interacts most, has a high degree of influence on behaviour, and is therefore the most important figure in the infant's early life. However, it was subsequently demonstrated that the amount of time the mother and infant spend together is not necessarily the best indicator of the closeness of the mother–child relationship or of the type of interaction between them, the more important issue being the quality of the interaction independently of the time spent together. Studies by Brofenbrenner (1975), Clarke-Stewart (1973), and Schaffer and Emerson (1964) have shown that the degree of interaction between mother and infant can be very low, even when the mother is in the same room or actually carrying the infant round with her, that daily separations due to the mother working do not *per se* cause any lessening of the infant's attachment to his mother, and that the quality of the interaction and the sensitivity of the mother to her infant's behaviour are the most important factors in early attachment. This concept of the quality of interaction and sensitivity to the infant's behaviour has also been demonstrated with fathers. Newson and Newson (1963) and Lamb (1975) showed that many fathers are highly accessible to their young children when they are at home and that, at least for some infants, a high degree of interaction with the father is possible and enjoyable, even when the time spent together is limited. Lamb also stressed that many fathers do not interact with their young offspring at all but, when they do, early attachment to the father does occur and a relationship with the infant is established. In his study of fathers and eight-month-old and two-year-old children, Lamb (1976) observed that the nature of the infant's relationship with his father was often different from that with his mother, the father being regarded more as a person to play with; two-year-old children were more likely to initiate play with the father than with the mother. This behaviour apparently stems from the fact that in infancy the mother is more likely to pick the child up to perform care-giving tasks than to play, whereas the reverse is true of fathers.

The relationship between father and child, as opposed to father and infant, has been the source of much research during the 1970s, notably by Biller (1971, 1974), who showed that an affectionate father–child relationship promotes the development of personality and sex roles: the absence of a father or inadequate fathering can seriously impair children's abilities to interact normally with members of both sexes in later life. Radin (1972) and Jordan et al. (1975) have indicated that a father's attitudes and nurturing behaviour can influence the cognitive development of his children and that this influence is stronger for boys than for girls. Here also the absence of a father during the early years can interfere with cognitive development, although the effects of this are complicated by many variables such as the reason for absence, the family composition and structure, and socio-economic status (Pederson et al., 1973; Blanchard and Biller, 1971).

In this area of child-rearing, as in most others, social class differences exist in both the time available and the type of involvement fathers have with their children. In general, middle class fathers have been shown to be more involved with child-rearing than lower class fathers (Lynn, 1974) and middle class wives have expressed different views of their husbands' role in the family from lower class wives (Kohn and Carroll 1960). Similarly, lower class fathers have been shown to be more authoritarian and to demand obedience and conformity from their children, whereas middle class fathers are more likely to assume a teaching role and generally to have a greater influence over family life (Benson, 1968; Freeberg and Payne, 1967; Hess and Torney, 1967).

These social class differences are not always cultural, as has been discussed in reference to the Newsons' study of children in Nottingham (Newson and Newson, 1968), when it was pointed out that the time available for a father to spend with the children will vary according to his working hours, especially if he is on shift work, away overnight or working away from home for long periods. While middle class fathers are more likely to work a regular eight-hour day and are therefore theoretically better able to plan the time they spend with their children, it is this group also who are more likely to be away on business overnight or for a few days at a time, thus making their time spent at home comparable to that of, for example, long-distance lorry drivers or fishermen. Similarly, a shift worker will only work 'unsocial' hours some of the time and may frequently be at home with his children during the day. If a wife also works, the hours she spends working may result in her husband taking care of the children for at least some of the time she is absent.

Finally, the type of relationship between the husband and wife must be considered when investigating the role of the father in child-rearing. As long ago as 1944, Baruch and Wilcox showed that marital conflict can interfere with the personality development of boys and girls. More recently, Block *et al.* (1973) have shown that the best adjusted adults are those who in childhood had warm relationships with effective mothers and fathers in the context of a happy marriage.

In summary, while the importance of the early bond between mother and infant remains undisputed, the influence of the father and of the marital relationship on the child's future emotional, psychological, behavioural, and intellectual development is less certain but cannot be discounted. One of the hypotheses in this survey is that early attachment between father and infant will lead to a productive relationship between them, giving the child additional support to that received from his mother in his intellectual and behavioural development.

To assess the type of relationship between husband and wife and the degree of involvement the father had with the study child, the women were asked the following questions in the hospital interviews:

To what extent they had discussed child-rearing, discipline, and contraception with their husbands

How much they expected their husbands to participate in certain tasks required in the care of the baby—feeding, changing, bathing, and getting to sleep

To what extent they expected their husbands to play with the baby and take him out alone

The amount of time they anticipated their husbands being able to spend with the baby each week

Significantly more control parents than LBW parents had discussed child-rearing and contraception but not problems of discipline (see Table 4.14). Control mothers also expected their husbands to spend more time with the baby and to share rather more in tasks concerning the baby. While these latter differences were not significant, it is noteworthy that to none of the questions did the LBW mothers present higher expectations of their husband's participation.

The pattern of intercorrelations (see Appendix, page 88) suggests a tighter picture. Thus, the three discussion variables—child-rearing, discipline, and contraception—all correlate positively and significantly with each other and two (child-rearing and discipline) correlate significantly with expectations for the husband to participate in changing, bathing, and getting the baby to sleep and with the amount of time husbands were expected to spend with the baby and his help in general. Similarly, the expectations for husband participa-

Table 4.14   Topics discussed by wife with husband

Topic	LBW %	Control %	p
Child-rearing*			
Yes	74.3	85.7	0.025
No	25.7	14.3	
Contraception†			
Yes	73.9	87.7	
No	20.0	10.0	
'Leave it to husband'	2.3	—	0.025
No comment	3.8	2.3	

* 140 pairs—excludes 3 LBW who were separated and their controls
† 130 pairs—12 women had been sterilized including 2 matched pairs and an additional 5 LBW and 3 control mothers; therefore, 10 further pairs have been excluded

tion variables intercorrelate positively (although only slightly so) with the amount of time the husbands were expected to spend with the baby.

The key variables in the pattern of intercorrelations appear to be the discussion variables (which report what has already occurred between the couple) rather than the expectations of participation (which report the wife's prediction of what might happen). However, one should distinguish between aspects of husband's participation which are essential and unavoidable, such as changing the baby and helping to get the baby to sleep, and those which, while essential, can be avoided by the husband.

A composite index has therefore been constructed by adding together the ranked scores obtained in response to the following questions about the role of the husband:

Amount of discussion of discipline with husband
Amount of discussion of child-rearing with husband
Amount of discussion of contraception with husband
Expectation of participation of husband in nappy changing
Expectation of help from husband in getting baby to sleep

This index of the *expected participation by the husband* can have values from 5

Table 4.15   Index of expected participation by husband: distribution in LBW and control groups

	9 and under	9.5–10.5	11–11.5	12–12.5	13–13.5	14 and over	Total
LBW	35	18	16	20	21	33	143
Controls	16	17	19	25	22	44	143
Total	51	35	35	45	43	77	286

Table 4.16 Index of expected participation by husband according to (a) mother's age and parity and (b) separately according to social class

(a)

	Mother's age							
	Under 25				25 and over			
	Index			Total	Index			Total
	10.5 and under	11–12.5	13 and over		10.5 and under	11–12.5	13 and over	
Primiparae								
LBW	19	16	18	53	4	6	10	20
Controls	14	17	31	62	1	6	4	11
Total	33	33	49	115	5	12	14	31
Multiparae								
LBW	10	5	12	27	20	9	14	43
Controls	3	11	14	28	15	10	17	42
Total	13	16	26	55	35	19	31	85

(b)

	Social Class											
	I–IIIa				IIIb				IV–V			
	Index			Total	Index			Total	Index			Total
	10.5 and under	11–12.5	13 and over		10.5 and under	11–12.5	13 and over		10.5 and under	11–12.5	13 and over	
LBW	3	7	23	33	26	9	16	51	24	20	15	59
Controls	3	8	22	33	17	14	23	54	13	22	21	56
Total	6	15	45	66	43	23	39	105	37	42	36	115

to 18. It is distributed in the study population and between LBW and controls as shown in Table 4.15. For the purposes of further analysis, the index is grouped in three categories (up to 10.5 corresponding to a low level of participation, between 11 and 12.5 corresponding to an average level of participation, and 13 or more corresponding to an involved father). With this grouping the differences between the LBW and controls is significant (χ^2 = 6.65, p <0.036). The breakdown according to mother's age and parity and separately according to social class is given in Table 4.16. It can be seen that while all the tables consistently show a trend of low expected involvement on the part of the LBW fathers as against relatively high expected involvement from the control fathers, the differences are only significant in respect of young multiparous mothers (see Table 4.7).

It appears, therefore, that in LBW families the husband is a more remote figure both practically and in terms of discussing the issues involved in bearing and raising a child, while in control families the husband is more likely to be involved both in discussing child-rearing and helping with the child.

Role rehearsal and planning for motherhood

The literature discussed earlier in relation to controlling and fatalistic orientations suggested planning and anticipation of future events as a characteristic of middle class behaviour. While this dimension has already been incorporated into the composite index of expectations to influence the child it seemed possible that it might also apply to planning for motherhood. Questions relevant to this issue in the sociological interview related to:

The reading of literature provided by the clinic
The use of other sources of information including published material as well
    as discussions with husbands, other relatives, and friends on child-rearing,
    weaning, potting, and general child development
The cessation of smoking during pregnancy
Deliberate changes of diet during pregnancy
The performance of antenatal relaxation exercises

Of all the items discussed in this section, only one showed a statistically significant difference between LBW and control mothers, namely the person(s) with whom the mother had had most discussion about child-rearing. More control mothers named their husband whereas LBW mothers were more likely to keep their own counsel or mention professionals. This significant difference applied overall and independently to primiparae and multiparae.

There were, however, pronounced differences between primiparae and multiparae: primiparous women practised much more role preparation and made more use of external sources of advice (see Table 4.17). Indeed, some of the questions may not have been very pertinent for multiparae. Therefore, we

Table 4.17   Behaviour during pregnancy

| | Primiparae 73 pairs | | Multiparae 70 pairs | | All 143 pairs | |
	LBW %	Control %	LBW %	Control %	LBW %	Control %
Antenatal Exercises Performed						
Yes	50.7	64.4	2.9	11.4	27.3	38.5
No	49.3	35.6	97.1	88.6	72.7	61.5
p	0.132		0.101		0.059	
Discussed most with						
No-one	8.2	1.4	20.0	7.1	14.0	4.2
Husband	32.9	52.0	30.0	38.6	31.5	45.5
Other rel. and friends	57.5	46.6	42.9	52.9	50.3	49.6
Professionals	1.4	—	7.1	—	4.2	—
Not stated	—	—	—	1.4	—	0.7
p	0.036		0.019		0.001	

shall be paying especial attention to the differences between the patterns observed for primiparae and multiparae.

The pattern of intercorrelations presented in the Appendix (page 88) suggests that the main linking variables in this group relate to the activity and initiative of the mother, such as whether she practised antenatal exercises, read beyond the literature supplied by the clinic, and changed her pattern of smoking during pregnancy. However, the extent to which she sought advice is also an important discriminator between LBW mothers, who relied more on themselves, and controls, who tended to seek advice from relatives and friends.

A composite index has been constructed by adding together the ranked scores obtained in response to three questions relating to the different stages of childbearing and raising:

Whether the mother practised antenatal exercises
Person talked to most about child-rearing ranked as any/none
Sources of advice on child development ranked as any/none

Table 4.18   Index of role preparation for motherhood: distribution in LBW and control groups

	3–3.5	4	4.5	5	5.5	6	Total
LBW	15	40	29	25	18	16	143
Controls	4	42	22	24	28	23	143
Total	19	82	51	49	46	39	286

Table 4.19 Index of role preparation for motherhood analysed according to (a) mother's age and parity and (b) separately according to social class

(a)

	Mother's age							
	Under 25				25 and over			
	4 and under	Index 4.5–5	over 5	Total	4 and under	Index 4.5–5	over 5	Total
Primiparae								
LBW	3	28	22	53	1	7	12	20
Controls	0	25	37	62	0	2	9	11
Total	3	53	59	115	1	9	21	31
Multiparae								
LBW	15	12	0	27	36	7	0	43
Controls	19	6	3	28	27	13	2	42
Total	34	18	3	55	63	20	2	85

(b)

	Social Class											
	I–IIIa				IIIb				IV–V			
	4 and under	Index 4.5–5	over 5	Total	4 and under	Index 4.5–5	over 5	Total	4 and under	Index 4.5–5	over 5	Total
LBW	5	9	19	33	27	17	7	51	23	28	8	59
Controls	6	7	20	33	20	18	16	54	20	21	15	56
Total	11	16	39	66	47	35	23	105	43	49	23	115

This index of the extent of *role preparation for motherhood* can have values between 3 and 6. It is distributed in the population and between cases and controls as shown in Table 4.18, which presents the score in six categories. However, for the purposes of further analysis, we clearly ought to combine these categories. The 'natural' division into three roughly equal groups is 4 and under, over 4 and up to 5, over 5. If this concatenation is made, the value of χ^2 is 4.84 which is not significant at the 5 per cent level ($p < 0.089$). As can be seen from Table 4.18, the problem is that, while there are two extreme groups—under 4 and 6 and over—the first is very small with only 19 members. But if we do compute χ^2 for the scores grouped in this way we obtain a value of $\chi^2 = 9.97$ which is highly significant ($p < 0.007$). While, therefore, Table 4.19 is presented according to the former breakdown, we shall also refer to this latter categorization into extreme groups.

The distributions of the values of the index when analysed according to mother's age and parity and separately according to social class are presented in Table 4.19. It can be seen that the only significant difference occurs with young primiparous mothers where those who score 4 or less are all LBW mothers and among those who score over 5 about 40 per cent are LBW mothers, while nearly 60 per cent are control mothers. No other differences reach formal significance although the p values for multiparous mothers are both low (0.065 and 0.079). Further, if we categorize in the alternative way suggested above, i.e. isolating the small group of 19 with the lowest scores, we find that there are significant differences with young multiparous mothers and with mothers married to husbands in Social Class IIIb.

It seems fair to conclude that there are significant differences in the amount of role preparation for motherhood between LBW and control groups even within age-parity or social class. The effect is strongest with young mothers.

Other differentiating features

Interviewer's assessments and mothers' 'don't know' responses

After each interview, the respondents were graded by the interviewer on three items—their vocabulary range, fluency of expression, and organization of thought. Table 4.20 shows the distribution of these subjective gradings, which were based on a scale of $1-9$. The control mothers had significantly higher gradings on all three items, indicating a wider range of vocabulary, greater fluency, and logic of thought. Because of the timing and place of the interviews the interviewers knew whether their respondents were LBW or control mothers.

In addition to the interviewer's assessments, the number of times each woman said 'I don't know' or, more colloquially, 'I dinna ken' to a question was counted. When reading the interviewer's reports, it was evident that some women had given little if any thought to some of the issues raised. The two sec-

Table 4.20 Interviewer's assessment at hospital interview (138 pairs)

		Score 1−3	4−6	7−9	p
Vocabulary range					
LBW	%	36.2	44.9	18.9	0.002
Control	%	17.4	58.7	23.9	
Fluency					
LBW	%	39.1	41.3	19.6	0.001
Control	%	15.2	56.5	28.3	
Logical thought					
LBW	%	38.4	44.2	17.4	0.003
Control	%	20.3	52.2	27.5	

tions of the interview where replies of 'dinna ken' were most frequent were, not surprisingly, expectations to influence the child's development and attitudes to behaviour training, which are both topics concerning more than the immediate future. The replies of the LBW and control mothers were not statistically different: but, whereas a similar proportion in both groups gave a specific answer to all five questions on expectation to influence child development, nearly twice as many LBW as control mothers replied that they did not know to at least one of the 11 questions on attitudes to behaviour training.

Further, when the cases are broken down into groups according to mother's age and parity and husband's social class, there are considerable differences.

These three interviewer assessments were highly intercorrelated, indicating that women who scored highly on one were very likely to score highly on the remaining two. Because of this a composite index has been constructed by adding together the three interviewers' ratings. This index of the *interviewers' assessments* can have values ranging from 3 to 30. It is distributed in the study population and between cases and controls as shown in Table 4.21. For the purposes of further analysis we have grouped this index into three categories: 11 and under, over 11 and under 17, and 17 and over. Using these, the differences between LBW and controls are highly significant, $\chi^2 = 13.83, p < 0.001$.

The distributions when broken down according to mother's age and parity, and separately according to social class, are presented in Table 4.22. It can be

Table 4.21 Index of interviewers' assessments: distribution in LBW and control groups

	8 and under	8.5−11	11.5−13.5	14−16.5	17−20.5	21 and over	Total
LBW	15	41	24	24	15	24	143
Controls	10	18	25	32	23	35	143
Total	25	59	49	56	38	59	286

Table 4.22   Index of interviewer's assessments of the mother (a) according to mother's age and parity and (b) separately according to social class

(a)

	Mother's age							
	Under 25				25 and over			
	Index			Total	Index			Total
	11 and under	11.5–16.5	17 and over		11 and under	11.5–16.5	17 and over	
Primiparae								
LBW	18	22	13	53	1	5	14	20
Controls	11	25	26	62	0	3	8	11
Total	29	47	39	115	1	8	22	31
Multiparae								
LBW	16	9	2	27	21	12	10	43
Controls	10	12	6	28	7	17	18	42
Total	26	21	8	55	28	29	28	85

(b)

	Social Class											
	I–IIIa				IIIb				IV–V			
	Index			Total	Index			Total	Index			Total
	11 and under	11.5–16.5	17 and over		11 and under	11.5–16.5	17 and over		11 and under	11.5–16.5	17 and over	
LBW	2	7	24	33	23	19	9	51	31	22	6	59
Controls	0	6	27	33	11	25	18	54	17	26	13	56
Total	2	13	51	66	34	44	27	105	48	48	19	115

seen that there are significant differences amongst older multiparous mothers and amongst mothers whose husbands are in Social Classes IIIb, and IV, V. Some of these differences are quite substantial: thus among older multiparous mothers half of the LBW mothers score 11 or less while five-sixths of the control mothers score more than 11, and among mothers with husbands in Social Class IIIb about two-fifths of LBW mothers score 11 or less while only one-fifth of control mothers score 11 or less.

It is clear that the interviewers distinguished between LBW and control mothers. They might have been influenced by foreknowledge but the differences are so sharp as to suggest a 'real' perceived difference between the mothers. Accordingly, we have retained this index for further analysis in Chapter 9.

Family planning

At the postnatal interview the women were asked about the number of children they wanted and their experiences and intentions in using contraception. The analysis of their replies is based on 140 matched pairs (71 primiparae and 69 multiparae) as three women were separated from their husbands and, with their matched pairs, have been excluded.

LBW mothers were significantly less likely to want more children but those who did want more wanted them more quickly than did the controls. The reasons given for their choice were highly significant, more LBW mothers giving medical and obstetric reasons compared with controls, the majority of whom gave financial reasons often coupled with statements about the interests of the child but expressions of disapproval of 'only' children.

More control mothers had discussed contraception with their husbands and were more likely to favour the pill or sheath in the future, whereas more LBW mothers favoured sterilization (15 LBW and 8 controls, in addition to the 7 LBW and 5 control mothers already sterilized). However, 3 LBW and 5 control mothers did not wish to be sterilized themselves but wanted their husbands to have a vasectomy. The differences support the general conclusion of the previous section in suggesting a stronger planning orientation and greater involvement of husbands (more typical of middle class behaviour) in the control group.

These data are not analysed in any further detail mainly because of their complexity, e.g. some women had been sterilized; medical and obstetric complications were involved in decisions; there were differences between primiparae and multiparae; and ordinal position was used in matching. An index could be constructed along the same lines as in previous sections but it would only be possible for a reduced number of pairs which would not be appropriate for subsequent use in Chapter 9.

CONCLUSION

The mothers of the LBW infants differed from their controls in their responses to 20 of the 75 questions and items of factual data covered in the sociological interview, whereas 4 different responses might have been expected at the 5 per cent level. In addition, the two groups differed socio-economically and in the interviewers' assessments, the control parents being at a socio-economic advantage over the LBW parents and receiving higher ratings for vocabulary, fluency of expression, and organization of thought. The variables which are statistically significant are indicated in Table 4.23.

However, the most important difference is that the mothers of LBW children are either very young or very old relative to both the controls and the general population of women giving birth during the study year. Because we have also argued that the aetiology of low birth weight is likely to be different for younger and older mothers, we have suggested that the mother's age should be treated as a basic classifying variable so that many of the analyses are carried out separately for young mothers and for older mothers.

Correlation analysis of the ranked replies to these questions reveals only a few relationships between variables, indicating that the areas where the LBW and control groups differ are on the whole independent of one another, although some relationships are present between types of recreational activity, expectations to influence and role preparation. The correlations between the recreational variables, expectations to influence school progress, the practice of antenatal exercises, advice on weaning, and whether child-rearing had been discussed with anyone in particular suggest that the control mothers may generally be more physically and mentally active than the LBW mothers, better informed, and more likely to work out a positive orientation to current and future activities and events.

Although the differences which exist between the LBW and control groups are quite small when taken individually, it proved possible to construct a series of indices which revealed rather larger differences between LBW and controls for seven groups of the variables. Two indices correspond to the socio-cultural environment as measured by the mobility and professional status and by the recreational activities of the parents, respectively; one indicated the extent to which parents expected to influence their child's development; one corresponded to the parents' attempts to train behaviour; one measured the extent to which the husband would be involved in the care of the baby; one indicated the amount of role rehearsal and preparation for motherhood undertaken prior to the birth; the final index was based on interviewer's assessment.

When the mothers are compared within sub-groups, defined by maternal age and parity and by the social class of the husband, it becomes clear that the major differences between LBW and controls in respect of these indices occur amongst young primiparous mothers and mothers whose husbands are in

Social Classes IV and V. The former result reinforces our view that it is important to treat young and old mothers separately; indeed, we should probably have used age as a matching variable. The latter result is either a function of the heterogeneity of Social Classes IV and V in occupational terms or suggests that, at least for some families, their life style is not so dependent on their occupational status.

In any event it is clear that, despite one-to-one matching by social class and by other class-related variables, the control group ranks higher on a series of dimensions likely to affect the development of children. However, there is little published work on the size of the potential impact of these influences on child development. To test how far outcome differences between LBW and control children at 10 years may be produced by these unplanned differences between the groups, the indices described in this chapter will be employed in the regression analyses of outcomes in Chapter 9.

APPENDIX TO CHAPTER 4

Ranking of replies and factual data from the hospital interviews

Rankings were derived from the categories of reply given by the mothers of the LBW and control babies during the interview in hospital after delivery, and were constructed after the data were collated.

The derived rankings are used for two purposes:

1. to calculate correlations between variables (see Table 4.23) and thus describe relationships between replies to different questions
2. to define numerically which categories may be regarded as the 'same' or 'similar' when comparing the replies of each pair of LBW—control mothers.

The basis for ranking categories of reply varied. The answers to some factual questions, e.g. age, duration of marriage, could be used directly whereas others, e.g. education or training, were ranked as were those on attitudes expectations, and practices by different criteria such as skill/achievement, frequency of contact/outings, degree of involvement/strictness, etc.

Some examples are given below and on page 90:

Social Class	Rank
I	6
II	5
IIIa	4
IIIb	3
IV	2
V	1

Table 4.23   Intercorrelations between the chosen variables in each block and with social class showing the p values for the test of differences between the LBW and control groups

Variable	Block intercorrelation			
	(1)	(2)	(3)	(4)
(1) Status of mother's last occupation	1.0	–	–	–
(2) House occupancy by security	0.42	1.0	–	–
(3) Husband's further training	0.28	0.13	1.0	–
(4) Mother's place of upbringing	−0.30	−0.09	−0.17	1.0
	(5)	(6)	(7)	(8)
(5) Usually go out in the evening with others	1.0	–	–	–
(6) First mentioned weekend activity is not TV	0.32	1.0	–	–
(7) Mention more than one weekend activity	0.16	0.34	1.0	–
(8) Mention more than one weekend activity in addition to TV and reading	0.15	0.20	0.24	1.0
	(9)	(10)	(11)	(12)
(9) Expect to influence crawling	1.0	–	–	–
(10) Expect to influence walking	0.43	1.0	–	–
(11) Expect to influence talking	0.21	0.37	1.0	–
(12) Expect to help child at school	0.21	0.14	0.31	1.0
(13) Opinion on heredity/environmental influence on school progress	0.07	0.11	0.16	0.15
	(14)	(15)	(16)	(17)
(14) Reaction to crying at night	1.0	–	–	–
(15) Daily routines	−0.22	1.0	–	–
(16) Reaction to thumb-sucking	0.14	−0.11	1.0	–
(17) Reaction to sucking other objects	−0.18	0.13	0.27	1.0
(18) Reaction to genital play	−0.07	0.02	0.29	0.23
(19) Reaction to child singing while mother has bad headache	−0.14	−0.05	0.12	0.16
(20) Reaction to child because friendly with undesirable	0.10	0.07	−0.10	0.08
(21) Reaction to child using bad language	0.15	−0.13	0.14	−0.11
	(22)	(23)	(24)	(25)
(22) Husband/wife discuss discipline	1.0	–	–	–
(23) Husband/wife discuss child-rearing	0.34	1.0	–	–
(24) Husband/wife disucss contraception	0.23	0.20	1.0	–
(25) Time husband will spend with baby	0.17	0.22	0.09	1.0
(26) Wife's expectation for husband's help with bathing baby	0.25	0.21	0.11	0.14
	(27)	(28)	(29)	
(27) Ante-natal exercises	1.0	–	–	
(28) Amount of reading on pregnancy/child-rearing	0.33	1.0	–	
(29) Advice on pottying	0.29	0.25	1.0	

Table 4.23 cont'd

				Correlation with social class	Significance of difference
				0.54	0.03
				0.17	N/S
				0.30	0.07
				−0.30	0.03
				0.20	0.06
				0.22	0.01
				0.10	0.01
				0.15	0.02
(13)					
—				0.18	N/S
—				0.13	N/S
—				0.15	N/S
—				−0.13	0.05
1.0				0.16	N/S
(18)	(19)	(20)	(21)		
—	—	—	—	−0.03	0.02
—	—	—	—	0.18	0.04
—	—	—	—	−0.17	0.05
—	—	—	—	−0.15	0.04
1.0	—	—	—	−0.29	N/S
−0.07	1.0	—	—	−0.12	0.03
0.12	0.17	1.0	—	0.21	N/S
0.09	0.16	0.23	1.0	0.13	0.02
(26)					
—				0.16	N/S
—				0.21	0.03
—				0.21	0.03
—				0.14	N/S
1.0				0.13	0.04
				0.27	0.06
				0.18	N/S
				0.13	0.10

Place of birth/upbringing	*Rank* (by distance from Aberdeen)
Aberdeen/north-east Scotland	4
Elsewhere in Scotland	3
Elsewhere in Britain	2
Overseas	1

Husband out alone	*Rank* (by frequency/week)
Very frequently, most nights	6
Mostly weekends	5
Regular once/week	4
Less than weekly	3
Infrequently/special occasions	2
Seldom/never	1

Reaction to baby sucking objects or to body play	*Rank* (by intervention/strictness)
Leave	1
Remove hand under certain conditions, e.g. if dirty	2
Distract, give dummy, rusk	3
Discourage/try to stop	4
Stop/remove hand	5
Smack	6

Details of the ranking of each variable are available from the authors.

Chapter 5

The Medical Study

J.I. CATER

The study sample comprised 149 LBW infants born in Aberdeen Maternity Hospital between 1 July 1969 and 31 December 1970 and 149 matched controls (see Chapter 3).

Many factors, including those relating to the mother and her experiences in pregnancy and delivery, and specific conditions of the newborn infant, are known to affect a child's subsequent development. For present purposes, these factors will be considered in five groups under two headings:

Maternal factors
Group I: Previous obstetric history
Group II: Medical conditions specific to pregnancy
Group III: Medical complications not specific to the pregnancy
Group IV: Maternal complications of delivery

Neonatal factors
Group V: Neonatal problems

MATERNAL FACTORS

Group I: Previous obstetric history

One crude measure of a woman's reproductive inefficiency is the number of pregnancies which did not result in a live child who survived the first postnatal week, i.e. the number of terminations, spontaneous abortions, stillbirths, and first week deaths. In the study sample, 57 LBW and 70 control mothers had no previous pregnancies. Of the remainder, the reproductive histories of the LBW mothers tended to be worse than those of the controls: in particular, the LBW mothers had had more spontaneous abortions and stillbirths.

Group II: Medical conditions specific to pregnancy

A number of medical conditions specific to pregnancy may contribute to later problems for the infant.

Pre-eclamptic toxaemia

Pre-eclamptic toxaemia (PET) is defined as an elevation of blood pressure occurring for the first time after the 25th week of pregnancy in association with oedema and proteinuria. It is associated with increased fetal mortality and morbidity and decreased rate of fetal growth.

The incidence of PET and hypertension in our LBW sample was almost twice that in the control group (35 LBW, 21 controls, $p < 0.05$).

Haemorrhage

The significance of haemorrhage depends in part upon its aetiology and whether it causes hypotension in either mother or fetus. Bleeding before 28 weeks is considered to be due to threatened abortion, episodes of which occurred significantly more frequently in the LBW group (42 LBW, 24 controls, $p < 0.025$). Haemorrhage after 28 weeks can be considered in three categories, viz. placenta praevia, abruptio placentae, and other antepartum haemorrhage of unknown origin. Two of these occurred only in LBW mothers (placenta praevia 5; abruptio placentae 3). Other forms of antepartum haemorrhage were significantly more frequent in the LBW than in the control group (LBW 23, controls 4, $p < 0.001$).

Cervical incompetence

Incompetence of the uterine cervix (neck of the womb) is a specific although infrequent cause of early pre-term birth. By inserting a Shirodker suture around the cervix, competence may be maintained, the suture being removed before delivery. This procedure had been carried out in 5 mothers of LBW babies but in none of the control mothers.

Group III: Medical complications not specific to the pregnancy

A number of medical disorders not specific to pregnancy may affect it adversely, for example, diabetes mellitus, urinary tract infection, anaemia, certain

Table 5.1 Frequency of medical complications not specific to the pregnancy

Condition	Number of mothers	
	LBW	Controls
Diabetes mellitus	3	2
Urinary tract infection	22	21
Anaemia	6	2
Gynaecological disorders	11	0
Respiratory infection	4	0
Other infections	21	14
Endocrine disorders	0	1
Heart disease	4	7
Tuberculosis	3	4
Nervous disorders	3	1

gynaecological disorders, respiratory and other infections, endocrine disorders, heart disease, and tuberculosis. Depression and other nervous conditions may also influence the mother's attitude to pregnancy, diet, and general health.

The incidence of these disorders in the LBW and control groups is shown in Table 5.1, which indicates that more LBW mothers suffered from anaemia, gynaecological disorders, and respiratory or other infections.

Group IV: Maternal complications of delivery

Premature rupture of the membranes

Premature rupture of the membranes constitutes a delicate balance of advantage and danger to the fetus. It is associated both with early delivery and its hazards and with increased risk of infection but, on the other hand, it may promote maturation of the pulmonary enzyme system responsible for the production of surfactant, thereby preventing idiopathic respiratory distress syndrome, a major cause of mortality in the pre-term infant. In this study, the membranes ruptured prematurely in the mothers of 26 LBW and 6 control infants.

Induction of labour

Induced labour carries a greater risk to the fetus than labour which occurs spontaneously. Nonetheless, initiation of labour in skilled hands for medical reasons can reduce mortality and morbidity. In Aberdeen in 1969 – 70, labour was often induced to avoid postmaturity and was carefully supervised by clinical means with frequent auscultation of the fetal heart : ultrasound techniques, scalp capillary blood sampling and fetal heart monitoring were little used as they were only at an early stage of development. Of the study sample, 43 LBW and 40 control mothers had induction of labour.

Presentation and delivery

Spontaneous vertex delivery has the lowest rate of complications associated with birth, all other methods of delivery carrying greater degrees of risk. Delivery was spontaneous in 62 per cent of the LBW mothers compared with 81 per cent of the control group. Assisted breech delivery, caesarean section, and forceps delivery were twice as frequent in the LBW group (assisted breech: 6 LBW and 3 controls; caesarean section: 23 LBW and 10 controls; forceps: 28 LBW and 15 controls).

Duration of labour

Prolonged labour, usually defined as labour in excess of 24 hours, is likely to have an adverse effect on the fetus. Nearly three times as many mothers of LBW babies had such a prolonged labour (25 LBW and 9 controls).

NEONATAL FACTORS

Before considering the neonatal problems of Group V, i.e. the various conditions of the infant which might have affected subsequent development, the general management and routine observation and measurement of the infants in the study will be described. A more detailed account has been recorded elsewhere (Cater, 1978).

Neonatal care

Infants requiring intensive care were transferred immediately from the delivery room to the adjoining special care baby unit (SCBU) where facilities included standard incubator care. Visiting of the baby was restricted to parents, to reduce the risk of cross-infection. Infants requiring respiratory support were ventilated with an East Radcliffe respirator (Tunstall *et al.*, 1968). Intravenous medication was usually given into the umbilical vein. Microsampling techniques were employed for determining levels of bilirubin, electrolytes, and glucose in the blood and for blood gas analysis. Plasma bilirubin levels were prevented from exceeding 20 mg% (342 μmol/l) by exchange transfusion.

The great majority of LBW babies were fed with half cream Cow and Gate milk (roller dried cow's milk with reduced fat content), while infants of normal weight were usually fed with full cream Cow and Gate milk. The policy was to start feeding LBW babies of normal growth at 12 hours of age, initially with 50 ml kg^{-1} body weight day^{-1} and reaching 150 ml kg^{-1} by the fifth day. LBW babies showing intra-uterine growth retardation were fed from 6 hours with the equivalent of 60 ml kg^{-1} day^{-1} reaching a full feed of 150 ml kg^{-1} by the fourth day. Intravenous feeding with 10 per cent dextrose by the umbilical vein was reserved for infants failing to tolerate oral feeds.

The duration of stay in a SCBU reflects a combination of admission policy, gestational age, birth weight, neonatal progress, and criteria for discharge. In our study, the LBW infants admitted to the SCBU spent up to 151 days there and 53 of them were kept for more than 28 days. Only 4 LBW infants were nursed beside their mothers (rooming in), compared with 148 of the control group. It should be realized that, at the time of the study, babies were usually kept in SCBUs far longer than is the present practice. The policy in Aberdeen in the 1960s was to admit all babies of birth weight 2500 g or less but by 1968 practice was beginning to change and heavier LBW babies were tending to be nursed beside their mothers in the postnatal wards. It seems likely that present admission and discharge policies based on clinical state, rate of weight increase above the minimum postnatal weight and quality of home circumstances (Davies *et al.*, 1979) will in future provide a better basis for assessing the relevance of duration of stay to long-term outcome.

Physical characteristics

General appearance

Each baby was described in terms of external physical features, state of nutrition, and any congenital malformation.

Birth weight

Before weighing, the baby was cleaned and dried and the umbilical cord was trimmed. The weight was recorded in grams using Avery baby scales, which were frequently checked and serviced. Table 5.2 shows the frequency distribu-

Table 5.2 Distribution of birth weight (149 LBW and matched controls)

LBW		Controls	
Grams	No. of infants	Grams	No. of infants
700 – 1000	2	2501 – 2750	16
1001 – 1250	3	2751 – 3000	24
1251 – 1500	8	3001 – 3250	31
1501 – 1750	12	3251 – 3500	32
1751 – 2000	21	3501 – 3750	21
2001 – 2250	29	3751 – 4000	20
2251 – 2500	74	4001 and over	5

tion of birth weights. Half of the LBW group weigh 2251 – 2500 g, which comes only marginally within the definition of LBW, while relatively few are of very low birthweight (1500 g and below). Few control infants are marginally above 2500 g (16 weigh 2750 g or less). It should be noted that the controls do not show the normal birth weight distribution because they are selected according to the criteria discussed in Chapter 3.

Gestational age

Gestational age at birth is considered to be the simplest indication of maturity in the newborn infant. In this study, an independent obstetrician (K.J. Dennis) calculated gestational age in days from the maternal history and recorded whether the information was considered to be certain or doubtful. The very low certainty rate (61 per cent LBW, 66 per cent controls) reflects the stringency of the definition as well as the increasing use of oral contraceptives in the years covered by the study. However, no significant difference was found in mean gestational age between 'certain' and 'doubtful' categories. Table 5.3 shows the frequency distribution of gestational age for the LBW group (range 27 – 41 weeks) and for controls (range 34 – 42 weeks). As would be expected the LBW group had a shorter mean gestational age than the controls (LBW 35.9 weeks, controls 39.7 weeks). It should be noted that age is calculated here in completed weeks, whereas for the purposes of a previous report (Cater, 1978) gestational age was expressed as incomplete weeks.

Gestational age indicates the chronological development of the fetus and is the yardstick against which morbidity patterns are commonly assessed: it is

Table 5.3 Distribution of gestational age in completed weeks (149 LBW and matched controls)

Gestational age (weeks)	LBW	Controls
31 and below	16	
32	7	–
33	12	–
34	6	1
35	18	–
36	14	–
37	17	4
38	24	20
39	23	30
40	8	60
41	4	29
42	–	5
Mean	35.9	39.7

therefore particularly important in any study of LBW infants. Estimation of gestational age based on the date of the last menstrual period is not always reliable and may be corroborated by various means: in this study, we used a simple and rapid clinical method based on external physical characteristics (Farr *et al.*, 1966a, b). A refinement of the simple use of gestational age in estimating intra-uterine growth retardation (IUGR) has been the use of weight for gestational age standards (Lubchenco *et al.*, 1963). In the present study, we used the centile standards of Thomson and his colleagues (1968), by which birth weight is corrected for the child's sex, maternal height, and pregnancy number. However, these standards are only applicable to children of gestational age of 32 weeks and over, since this is the lower limit set by the charts. The LBW sample was divided into five groups on the basis of both birthweight centile position and gestational age. Infants below 32 weeks were termed 'very premature'; those of less than 37 weeks, 'premature'; and those of 37 or more weeks, 'term'. (The word 'premature' has largely been dropped in favour of 'pre-term' but we have retained it here for the purpose of this classification.)

Our five groups are thus defined:

1. *Very premature*: all LBW infants with gestational age of less than 32 weeks ($N = 16$).
2. *Growth retarded premature*: all LBW infants on or below the 10th centile with gestational age of 32 weeks and above but less than 37 weeks ($N = 16$).
3. *Premature*: all LBW infants above the 10th centile with gestational age of 32 weeks and above but less than 37 weeks ($N = 41$).
4. *Growth retarded*: all LBW infants below the 10th centile with gestational age of 37 weeks or more ($N = 69$).
5. *Small normal*: all LBW infants above the 10th centile with gestational age of 37 weeks or more ($N = 7$).

Anthropometric measurements

Measurements were made in triplicate of the occipito-frontal circumference, crown – heel length and crown – rump length in all babies. For crown – heel length, the infant was placed in a specially designed measuring box, the head being held by an assistant against a fixed headboard. The examiner straightened the lower limbs at the knees, brought the footboard into position and made the measurement.

Postnatal progress

Clinical events

Details of clinical events were routinely recorded. Information on the occurrence of apnoeic and cyanotic attacks, convulsions, infections, respiratory distress syndrome, oedema, and other disease states and their subsequent management was obtained from these routine records.

Laboratory data

Measurements were made to detect biochemical changes that might have a damaging effect on subsequent development of the child. Those chosen were changes in the levels of blood glucose and serum bilirubin and in the packed cell volume of the blood. During the first 72 hours, 7 pre-feed values for blood glucose were obtained for LBW infants (at 10.30 am, 4.30 pm, and 10.30 pm) and 3 for control infants (at 1 pm). Capillary blood was obtained by stabbing a warmed heel and was immediately precipitated according to the method of Morley *et al.* (1968). Samples refrigerated for more than 48 hours showed no significant deterioration, so analysis was carried out during the normal working week. In urgent clinical situations, the dextrostix test was used and the result confirmed later by the method of Hoffman (1937), which was used routinely at that time.

Samples for serum bilirubin estimation were obtained when clinically necessary. Bilirubin levels in LBW babies were routinely recorded on the fifth day, even in those with little or no jaundice. Serum bilirubin was measured in the hospital laboratory by a standard method (O'Hagan *et al.*, 1957).

Packed cell volume was estimated in capillary blood in duplicate, using the Hawksley microhaematocrit.

Group V: Neonatal problems

Fetal distress

Fetal distress may presage both initial neonatal and long-term clinical and neurological problems. Difficulty arises in defining its severity and duration: at the time of the study, clinical methods, mainly auscultation of the fetal heart, were used and biochemical and ECG monitoring of the fetus was only introduced later.

Meconium staining of the liquor amnii and changes in fetal heart rate (evidence of fetal distress) were noted in 15 LBW and 18 control infants and 54 LBW and 33 controls, respectively.

Low Apgar score

The changes of asphyxia are intensified when respiration fails to start. They are falling oxygen levels, rising carbon dioxide levels, and increasing acidity of the blood. The Apgar Score (Apgar, 1953) is now widely used as an indication of the degree of asphyxia and is based on five clinical features, namely, skin colour, heart rate, respiratory pattern, muscle tone, and response to stimuli. Drage and Berendes (1966) reported that infants with low scores (0 – 1) at 1 and 5 minutes after birth had neonatal mortality rates of 23 per cent and 49 per cent, respectively. Results from the American collaborative study (Drage *et al.*, 1966) show that the 5 minute Apgar score is the best indicator of neurological abnormality. Though it is thus a useful clinical tool, its association with permanent neurological damage is not particularly strong, as the score may only reflect the infant's condition during a short period of time around birth.

Apgar scores were routinely recorded at 1 and 5 minutes after birth. Scores were obtained for all control babies but not for one LBW baby born before arrival at hospital: for another LBW baby, born in the ambulance on the way to hospital, only a 5 minute score was obtained. Apgar scores of 3 or less at 1 minute were recorded in 36 LBW infants and 7 controls while at 5 minutes, 9 LBW and 1 control infant scored 5 or less. Low Apgar scores were rather more frequent in the LBW group than would be expected today due to current trends in obstetric care, which are towards avoidance of the use of pethidine and similar drugs in the management of early delivery.

Apnoea/cyanosis

Apnoea has been defined as 'a non-breathing interval longer than an infant can tolerate without bradycardia and cyanosis'. This may be 20 seconds for a larger pre-term infant and as short as 5 seconds in a small one (Dailly *et al.*, 1969). Before cardiorespiratory monitors were widely used, difficulty was often experienced in distinguishing cyanotic attacks from truly apnoeic periods. Cyanosis might herald the beginning of an apnoeic attack or be associated with a purely mechanical problem such as choking on a plug of mucus.

Of the LBW babies, 4 suffered apnoea attacks only, 5 had cyanosis only, and 4 had both conditions. Where the distinction between apnoea and cyanosis was difficult the baby was defined as being 'off colour' and a further 13 LBW infants were included in this category. All three items were combined in a composite category (cyanotic index) in which 26 LBW infants were included.

Convulsions

Convulsions in the newborn period are associated with an increased incidence of neurological abnormality at follow-up. However, the prognosis depends to a considerable extent on the aetiology. For example, hypocalcaemic convulsions carry a more favourable outlook than fits caused by intracranial haemorrhage or congenital structural anomalies.

Convulsions were recorded in 4 LBW infants, 2 of whom had hypoglycaemia, and in 1 control infant.

Respiratory distress syndrome

Respiratory distress in the newborn period results from a wide variety of clinical conditions, including congenital malformation, pneumonia, pneumothorax, idiopathic respiratory distress syndrome (immaturity of the pulmonary enzyme system), transient tachypnoea (delayed clearing of fluid from the lungs) and cardiac and cerebral disorders. Idiopathic respiratory distress syndrome accounted for 15 per cent of early neonatal deaths in the British Perinatal Mortality Survey (Butler and Bonham, 1963). With improvement in understanding and therapeutic techniques, such as the use of continuous positive airway pressure (Gregory *et al.*, 1971), mortality seems to have been reduced. In this study, the respiratory distress syndrome was held to include idiopathic respiratory distress, transient tachypnoea, and infection. In theory, the distinction between these is clear but clinical differentiation is often difficult. In all, 32 LBW infants were considered to have this syndrome, as indicated by a positive Silverman Score. This is an index of respiratory distress based on allocating 0, 1 or 2 points to each of five features, viz. the degree of retraction of the upper chest, lower chest, and xiphoid process; dilatation of the nostrils; and expiratory grunt. A total score of 0 indicates no respiratory distress, while 10 indicates very severe distress (Silverman, 1961). The 32 LBW infants with respiratory distress had scores from 2 to 7.

Mechanical ventilation

Mechanical ventilation was used on two indications—severe repeated apnoeic attacks and respiratory failure due to the respiratory distress syndrome. It was required by 3 LBW infants (1 suffering from a combination of respiratory distress syndrome and apnoea and 2 with apnoeic attacks) and by none of the controls. The method was that described by Tunstall *et al.* (1968).

Exchange transfusion

Exchange transfusion was carried out in jaundiced babies with a sufficiently high level of plasma bilirubin to be at risk of deafness and/or athetoid cerebral palsy, the object being to keep the level of indirect-reacting bilirubin below 20 mg 100 ml^{-1} (342 μmol l^{-1}).

Four LBW babies received a total of 5 exchange transfusions for hyperbilirubinaemia. A further 2 babies received 3 exchange transfusions to control severe Rhesus iso-immunization: their bilirubin levels did not exceed 20 mg% (342 μmol l^{-1}).

Glucose therapy

Hypoglycaemia is defined as a blood glucose valve below 20 mg 100 ml^{-1} (1.1 mmol l^{-1}) in LBW infants and 30 mg 100 ml^{-1} (1.7 mmol l^{-1}) in heavier babies

(Cornblath *et al.*, 1966). According to this criterion, 9 LBW infants and 1 control had hypoglycaemia.

Solutions of 10 per cent glucose were routinely infused in ill and very preterm infants and their use affords one indication of the baby's condition: 31 LBW infants and 1 control required this therapy.

Solutions of 25 per cent glucose were administered therapeutically to 2 LBW babies demonstrating clinical and/or biochemical signs of hypoglycaemia, and to none of the control infants.

Bicarbonate therapy

In the late 1960s and early 1970s, sodium bicarbonate was widely used to correct acid-base imbalance of babies with severe respiratory distress syndrome (Usher, 1963). Bicarbonate is now rarely employed due to the increasing use of ventilators and continuous positive airway pressure in infants with severe respiratory distress and the realization that sodium bicarbonate has an association with intraventricular haemorrhage (Simmons *et al.*, 1974). Bicarbonate therapy was administered to 20 of the LBW infants and none of the control infants in this study.

Blood pressure

There is a known association between low blood pressure and subsequent clinical problems. Hall and Oliver (1971) reported on 37 infants with blood pressure less than 40 cm water on admission: of the 18 who were treated 5 survived whereas the 19 untreated infants all died. It is also well known that LBW babies have lower blood pressures than those of normal birth weight. In this study, systolic blood pressure was routinely recorded between 12 and 36 hours after birth, using the simple pulse indicator described by Ashworth *et al.* (1959). The mean value for the control infants was 69.1 mmHg (S.D. 6.2) which is significantly higher ($p < 0.001$) than for the LBW infants (60.6 mmHg, S.D. 8.9).

MATERNAL AND NEONATAL INDICES

The five groups of factors discussed above provided the basis for the construction of five indices which were intended to give an indication of the risk to the infant.

1. *Previous obstetric history index*   The score given was the total number of failed pregnancies for each mother who had had at least one previous pregnancy, account being taken of women in their first pregnancy.
2. *Medical conditions specific to pregnancy index*   This index was derived by the summation of the number of conditions specific to pregnancy which each woman experienced during this pregnancy.

3. *Medical complications not specific to the pregnancy index*   The score for this index was the summation of the number of general medical conditions each woman experienced during this pregnancy.

4. *Maternal complications of delivery index*   This index was derived by allocating one point to each of the following:

(a) Abnormal presentation
(b) Premature rupture of the membranes
(c) Prolonged labour
(d) Induction.

The type of delivery was accorded 0–2 points depending on the degree of risk:

(a) vertex and elective caesarean section were given a score of 0;
(b) Other caesarean section and low forceps delivery, 1 point
(c) High forceps and assisted breech delivery, 2 points.

These scores were then added together to form the total.

5. *Neonatal problems index*   Scores were derived by allocating one point for each of the following and adding them together:

(a) Mechanical ventilation
(b) Exchange transfusion (regardless of number)
(c) Respiratory distress syndrome;
(d) Convulsions
(e) Apnoeic attacks (any number)
(f) Systolic blood pressure below 40
(g) Evidence of fetal distress
(h) Oedema (excluding orbital)
(i) 10 per cent glucose therapy
(j) 25 per cent glucose therapy
(k) Bicarbonate therapy
(l) Apgar score at 1 minute of 3 or less and Apgar score at 5 minutes of 5 or less.

From Table 5.4 it is apparent that for each of the indices the LBW group is at a disadvantage. The difference is particularly striking in the case of medical conditions specific to pregnancy, complications of delivery and neonatal problems. Table 5.5 indicates the extent to which LBW infants in the lower birth weight range (under 2000 g) were disproportionately disadvantaged in relation to neonatal problems.

Table 5.6 shows that the five birth weight centile/gestational age groups have incurred different degrees of risk. The basis for the Table is that most of the control group score 0 or 1 on four indices and up to 2 for the fifth (maternal complications of delivery), hence the cut-off points used. The 'very premature' infants had a considerable preponderance of neonatal problems but otherwise were only at fairly limited risk to complications of pregnancy: presumably some potential risks were not incurred due to the short gestation and limited time in utero. The 'growth retarded prematures' had the highest proportion of mothers in their second or later pregnancy—87 per cent compared with 69 and 65 per

Table 5.4 Percentage distribution of scores in maternal and neonatal indices (149 LBW infants and matched controls)

Score	Previous obstetric history† LBW %	Control %	Medical conditions specific to pregnancy LBW %	Control %	Medical complications not specific to the pregnancy LBW %	Control %	Maternal complications of delivery LBW %	Control %	Neonatal problems LBW %	Control %
0	69	82	46	71	62	69	38	56	24	62
1	22	14	33	25	25	27	33	32	35	31
2	6	3	20	3	10	4	22	10	11	5
3+	3	1	1	1	3	–	7	2	30	2
p	0.097		<0.0001		0.036		0.001		<0.0001	

†Excluding the women who had had no previous pregnancy.

Table 5.5 Percentage distribution of scores in maternal and neonatal indices by weight of LBW infant (149 infants)

Score	Previous obstetric history† LBW ≤2000 g	LBW >2000 g	Medical conditions specific to pregnancy LBW ≤2000 g	LBW >2000 g	Medical complications not specific to the pregnancy LBW ≤2000 g	LBW >2000 g	complications of delivery LBW ≤2000 g	LBW >2000 g	Neonatal problems LBW ≤2000 g	LBW >2000 g
0	48	56	59	63	37	50	37	39	4	32
1	33	34	33	22	39	30	39	30	20	42
2	11	5	4	13	22	20	20	23	20	8
3+	8	5	4	2	2	0	4	8	56	18
p	0.557		0.234		0.224		0.666		<0.0001	

† Includes women in second or later pregnancy only.

Table 5.6 Percentage distribution of scores in maternal and neonatal indices by birth weight centile/gestational age groups (149 LBW infants)

	Very premature	Growth-retarded premature	Premature	Growth-retarded	Small normal
Number of infants	16	16	41	69	7
Previous obstetric history—% scoring 2+	6.2	21.0	14.6	3.0	0.0
Medical conditions specific to pregnancy—% scoring 2+	25.0	26.3	19.5	16.6	42.9
Medical complications not specific to the pregnancy—% scoring 2+	6.2	15.8	9.7	15.1	14.3
Maternal complications of delivery—% scoring 3+	0.0	0.0	4.8	10.6	14.3
Neonatal problems—% scoring 2+	81.2	47.4	53.7	26.6	0.0

cent in the 'very premature' and 'premature' groups, respectively, and 71 and 43 per cent in the 'growth retarded' and 'small normal' groups, respectively. Mothers in the 'growth retarded premature' group had relatively poor obstetric histories and the babies were also at some risk from their mothers' general health and conditions specific to pregnancy. Neonatal problems were fewer than in the 'very premature' group but were still significantly frequent. The 'premature' group also had an excess of neonatal problems. The 'growth retarded' infants had fewer neonatal problems but were at greater risk of delivery complications than any of the 'premature' groups of infants.

'Small normal' infants were similar to the 'growth retarded' group in relation to the mother's general health and delivery complications but seemed to be more at risk from specific pregnancy complications. However, the interpretation of these findings is doubtful as there were only seven infants in this group.

CONCLUSIONS

1. Mothers and infants in the LBW group were at a considerable disadvantage in comparison with their controls.
2. Lighter LBW infants had more neonatal problems than heavier ones, irrespective of maternal histories and experiences.
3. Five birth weight centile/gestational age groups were defined and used in the analysis of the data. From this it was concluded that the number of neonatal problems was in inverse proportion to the length of gestation and that LBW infants born at term were especially at risk from complications of delivery. The worst obstetric histories tended to be found in the 'premature' groups.
4. Infants born very early ('very premature') were at less risk from maternal illness than other groups of LBW infants.

Chapter 6

The Follow-Up Study: Tracing and Interviewing the Children

A. HEWITT

There are many problems in maintaining, or subsequently re-establishing, contact with the subjects of longitudinal research studies but no effort appears to have been made by research workers to pool information about records systems and tracing methods. Little attention is usually paid in research reports to the techniques used to locate the sample, even though the efficacy of these techniques largely determines the success of the follow-up study. In the light of this, it is hoped that this account of the tracing methods used in the Aberdeen LBW Study will prove of interest to research workers planning or engaged in comparable studies.

There were 298 children in the original Aberdeen LBW Study in 1969–70. One of the LBW babies died in infancy, and when the control child had been excluded, this left 296 children to be located for the follow-up in 1979–80. It was the task of the organizing secretary, who was employed on a half-time basis, to trace these children, obtain parental permission for them to take part in the follow-up, and arrange the interview programme for the medical officer and psychologist.

PRELIMINARIES: ACCESS TO RECORDS AND CO-OPERATION REQUIRED

It was assumed at the outset that the majority of the sample would still be living in Aberdeen or elsewhere in the Grampian Region, and that the greater part of the interviewing would take place within the Region.

105

The co-operation of the health authorities for the area had to be secured before the field work for the Study could begin. As the children were of school age and it was hoped to arrange for the medical examinations and the intelligence tests to be conducted in the schools, the approval and active support of the education authority was also a necessary prerequisite.

The Study first received the approval of the Director of Education for the Grampian Region, who agreed that the children could be interviewed in the schools. Following upon this, the organizing secretary was given permission to make use of the records system maintained by the Chief School Welfare Officer and his staff. Permission was also given to make direct contact with other education offices in the Region when necessary, to trace the children, and to make direct contact with the schools to arrange the interview programme and to confirm the whereabouts of children.

The Aberdeen LBW Study also received the approval of the Grampian Health Board, the community medicine specialist responsible for the operation of the School Health Service, and the General Practice Sub-committee of the Board, which undertook to notify all general practitioners in the area about the Study. Permission was given at the outset to make use of records held by the Community Health Division for tracing purposes and later, as the tracing process evolved, the organizing secretary was given access to the nominal index of patients registered with general practitioners in the area, which is maintained by the Primary Care Registration section of the Grampian Health Board. Before the field work commenced, access was also granted to the records held in the Royal Aberdeen Children's Hospital and the Aberdeen Maternity Hospital.

TRACING THE SAMPLE: THE BACKGROUND

When the field work began in July 1979, the organizing secretary thus had access to various educational and medical records systems, but her remit to locate 296 children did not prescribe the procedure to be adopted. A limited amount of advice was available, but essentially she had to devise her own tracing methods by a system of trial and error as the work proceeded. The principal justification of the laborious, time-consuming, and sometimes unorthodox methods employed to trace the Aberdeen LBW Study sample lies in their results, for no fewer than 290 of the 296 children were traced (98 per cent). Of the remaining six children, one is known to be living abroad and one in the Grampian Region with highly peripatetic parents; the mother of a third is known to have re-married and 'gone away South', leaving only three about whom it was impossible to discover any information.

A general philosophy relating to both the tracing procedures and the subsequent interviewing evolved quite rapidly once the field work began. Though it was clear from the start that success would be dependent in part on the active co-operation of others—in particular the parents, the children themselves, and the staffs of the schools and records departments—it also became apparent that the more independently the Study team could operate within this framework of support, the more successful would be their efforts. The follow-up study was therefore designed to cause the minimum of inconvenience to other people.

At the beginning of the field work the information possessed by the organizing secretary was each child's Christian name and surname at birth, his date of birth, and the address at which the family was living when the child was born, which were listed in a register retained from the first phase of the Study in 1969 – 70. The child's unit number of the Royal Aberdeen Children's Hospital records and the mother's unit number in the Aberdeen Maternity Hospital records were also available. There had been a general intent to follow up the children at some unspecified date in the future and consequently an effort had been made for a few years to keep in touch with the families. Birthday cards were sent out to the children until their fourth birthday and a few families had notified changes of address.

An investigation had also been conducted in 1975 into the number of times the children in the LBW Study had attended the Accident and Emergency Department of the Royal Aberdeen Children's Hospital and as a result a number of changes of address had been recorded. It was not explicitly stated in the register that all the addresses which had not been changed had been found to be correct, though the inference was that they had. Addresses were sometimes recorded for families who had left Aberdeen, but sometimes not. In some cases the date on which a family had changed address was noted, and the latest of these was mid-October 1974. No subsequent changes had been recorded, so at the beginning of the follow-up all the addresses were at least four and a half years old. No telephone numbers had been recorded at any point. Useful biographical information about the families, such as the full names of both parents, could be extracted from the interview schedules conducted with the mothers soon after birth of the infants in 1969 – 70. These interview schedules were available at the Institute of Medical Sociology, where the LBW Study had its office, but in practice the organizing secretary only referred to them to gather additional information about the families of children who posed a tracing problem.

The children in the LBW Study were born over an eighteen-month period from July 1969 to December 1970, and it was a formulated aim of the follow-up study to interview them within a three-week margin on either side of their tenth birthday, if possible. This meant that interviewing, like the births, had to take place over an eighteen-month period. This requirement influenced the procedures adopted for tracing the sample, because it meant that enough children had always to be ready traced and recruited into the follow-up to maintain a continuous interview programme for the medical officer and the psychologist. In practice, the organizing secretary traced the children chronologically in two-or three-month cohorts, and aimed always to keep about three months ahead of the interviewers. It was found most practicable to trace about 40 children at a time, and the number involved determined whether a tracing group consisted of children born over a two-month or a three-month period. Once the first group (39 children born in July, August, and September 1969) had been traced, the procedure was to procure parental permission for them to take part, and set up an interview programme for them during July, August and September 1979, while at the same time work was in hand on tracing the next group.

Certain practical limitations on the usefulness of the major records systems used in tracing the sample were encountered. In the case of the educational records, the problems arose from administrative inconsistencies which stemmed from the major reorganization of local government which took place in Scotland in 1975. Under the old system, the city of Aberdeen was a local authority in its own right, and Aberdeen City Council had its own Department of Education headed by a Director of Education. When local government was reorganized on a regional basis, following the passage of the Local Government (Scotland) Act in 1973, the city boundaries were extended to take in sizeable suburban areas on its outskirts, which had previously been administered by the counties of Aberdeenshire and Kincardineshire. The extended city is now known in local government terms as the Aberdeen District, and is one of five administrative districts within the Grampian Region. Education is one of the functions for which the Region is responsible, and it is administered by the Grampian Regional Council's Education Department. Records systems, however, have not necessarily been brought into line with the new administrative arrangements. The records kept by the School Welfare section, the principal educational records system used in tracing the LBW Study sample, still referred only to children in the 'old' city of Aberdeen. No comparable system covered school pupils in the large housing areas incorporated into the Aberdeen District in 1975, or pupils in the rest of the Grampian Region.

An additional complication was the fact that, although the administrative boundaries of the Grampian Health Board area coincide with those of the Grampian Region, the boundaries of the sub-divisions within the two do not. However, the nominal index of patients maintained by the Primary Care Registration section, which was the principal system of records used for tracing the children, did cover the whole of the Grampian Health Board area. Its chief limitation was that, because of the mobility of its population and the frequency with which changes in name and status occur, the records were not always accurate or up-to-date.

Changes in the family unit due to bereavement, separation, divorce, and re-marriage inevitably add to the complexity of tracing a sample for a longitudinal research study. Since there was no specific sociological component to the follow-up in the Aberdeen LBW Study, the staff had no formal means of measuring the incidence of such events. In the course of tracing the children, however, and in subsequent conversation with them, domestic events of this kind frequently came to light. They are known to have affected a minimum of 32 LBW and 20 control children (Table 6.1). The fact that the family circumstances of one-sixth of the children in the sample had altered over a ten-year period is an indication of the scale of the problem facing a records system such as that maintained by the Primary Care Registration section.

Table 6.1   Known family complications*

	LBW	Control	Total
Changed surname			
Mother and child	10[1]	7[1]	17[2]
Mother only	4	–	4
Parents known to be living apart	17	9	26
Child in care	2	3	5
Total	33	19	52
Parent dead			
Mother	2	–	2
Father	2	2	4
Total	4	2	6

* These are minimum figures. A number of other families are known to have been in difficulties, but no precise details were established.
( ) Remarried after bereavement.

It was against this background of practical and administrative difficulties that the 296 children in the LBW Study had to be located. When tracing a group of children, the organizing secretary set out with two aims: to ascertain the current home address of each child and to ascertain the primary school he was attending. The decision to conduct the interviewing in the schools, which was made for the benefit of the children and their parents, gave an additional dimension to the tracing problem, because two specific pieces of information had to be discovered rather than one.

There is no centralized register of all children in the Aberdeen area, let alone in the Grampian Region, which would have provided the information required. Educational records and medical information gathered about children by the School Health Service tends to be kept at the schools, and the school a child attends is largely determined by the address at which he lives. The school population in the Grampian Region is zoned, so that children living in a given area will go to a certain area primary school and then on to a certain secondary school. It is possible for children to be granted zoning exemptions on various grounds, and the children of Roman Catholic families have the option of attending one of the three Roman Catholic primary schools in Aberdeen rather than their area primary school. In addition, there are two private fee-paying schools for girls and one for boys in Aberdeen, which are not affected by zoning considerations. For the most part, however, a child's home address will determine the school he attends and, therefore, for the purpose of tracing the sample for the LBW Study, a current home address for each child was of paramount importance. (Government legislation since the time of writing entitles parents to choose their children's schools and the zoning system no longer operates in the Grampian Region.)

In tracing the children, many different techniques were used, but the majority of them (224) were found by way of two main records systems. The first was that maintained by the Grampian Regional Council's School Welfare Department, which carried out a range of welfare functions in relation to the school population in Aberdeen. The second was the nominal index of patients registered with general practitioners in the Grampian Health Board area, which is maintained by the Primary Care Department's Registration section. As an intermediate measure much use was also made of records on pre-school children dating back a decade, which were available at the Health Board's Community Health Division. The children traced by these means can be described as having been found by routine tracing methods (Table 6.2).

From the procedural point of view, with each group of children traced, it was necessary to concentrate initially on the majority who could be located through the basic procedures as here defined, so that letters about them could be sent

Table 6.2   Children located by routine tracing procedures

Date of birth	Routine procedure	No. of children
July – Sept. 1969	School Welfare alone	27
	School Welfare + phone calls to schools/education offices	5
October 1969 – April 1970	Community Health + School Welfare	75
	Community Health + phone calls to schools	12
	Community Health + School Welfare + phone calls to schools	4
May – December 1970	Primary Care Registration + School Welfare	73
	Primary Care Registration + phone calls to schools	28
	Using routine procedures: Total traced	224
	Untraced	72
	Total children in study	296

Table 6.3   Tracing groups and outcome

Children born	Total no.	Located by routine procedures	Tracing problems
1. July – Sept 1969	39	32	7
2. Oct – Nov 1969	41	32	9
3. Dec 1969 – Jan 1970	37	27	10
4. Feb – April 1970	50	32	18
5. May – June 1970	53	43	10
6. July – Sept 1970	45	35	10
7. Oct – Dec 1970	31	23	8
Total	296	224	72

out to parents and schools, and the interview programme kept on schedule. Only then was time available to concentrate on the tracing problems in the Study, who averaged 10 in each tracing group, and numbered 72 in all (Table 6.3).

THE ROUTINE TRACING

The first group of 39 children born in July, August, and September 1969, was traced primarily with the assistance of the staff of the School Welfare Department which, though administratively a section of Grampian Regional Council's Department of Education, still clearly reflected its roots in the pre-1975 organization of local government, when the city of Aberdeen had its own education department. The city had employed a team of school welfare officers, whose duty it was to act as links between home and school in cases where children were displaying behavioural problems at school, or playing truant from school. Each officer had responsibility in this respect for a secondary school in the city and the primary schools which sent children to it at age 11, and their work was dependent on a deep personal knowledge of a particular area of the city and its inhabitants. The department continued its work after the reorganization of local government, but the team of school welfare officers was not augmented to cover the extensive housing areas which came within the boundaries of the new Aberdeen District. The whereabouts of children who were known or thought to be living in these areas could not therefore be ascertained at the School Welfare Department.

Each officer maintained what was in essence a street census book of the area for which he was responsible, recording details of all the families with children of school age. These meticulously maintained, handwritten books gave the address of each such family, the name of the adult householder, and the names and dates of birth of all the children of school age, along with the name of the school they were attending. When a family left the area, the officer would normally record the address to which they were moving and, when a family came into the area, he would normally record the address from which they had come.

The books currently being maintained by the school welfare officers covered a school session, which in the Grampian Region runs from late August to early July. Books covering previous years, dating back as far as 1959 – 60, were stored in the department and could be consulted if necessary. Because all the books were organized on a geographical basis according to school zoning areas, it proved helpful if the list of children to be traced was also organized geographically on the basis of the last known addresses. It was then possible to check the appropriate school welfare officer's current book, to see if the family was still resident at the last known address. If they were not, it was possible to check back through the old books until a reference was found which indicated when they had moved, and where they had moved to. If the move was within the pre-1975 city boundaries, the address could then be counterchecked in whichever current book was appropriate. It would be recorded in the book whether the child was attending his local primary school, or had a zoning exemption to attend another school, or was a pupil at a special school for mentally and physically handicapped children, or at a Roman Catholic primary school, or at a private fee-paying school. The books sometimes gave an indication that a family had split up, or that a mother and/or her children were known by a name other than the one they were using ten years previously.

The School Welfare Department also had records dating back some years on children who had left city schools and moved away from the area, which sometimes, but not always, gave a specific forwarding address. It had information about zoning exemptions, about children in attendance at special schools and hospitals, and about children who had been taken into the care of the local authority, and were living with foster parents or in Children's Homes. The two clerical officers who staffed the School Welfare Department office had between them an impressive fund of accumulated knowledge about the school population of Aberdeen, knowledge that on occasion transcended anything that was written down anywhere. They were unfailingly helpful and during the course of the organizing secretary's first visit spent a great deal of time tracing the children and giving instructions on how to use the system. On subsequent visits the organizing secretary was able to do the bulk of the tracing herself, only asking the clerical officers for assistance when she had drawn a blank. They would than have recourse to files on children who had left the area and to various other files which might yield specific information about the whereabouts of a family at some given point in time, and so open up a new line of enquiry.

The somewhat paternalistic but highly efficient system operated by the School Welfare Department was of invaluable assistance in tracing the sample for the Aberdeen LBW Study. Its chief virtues were that it was up to date and highly accurate, and also provided a confirmed home address for the children and information about which school they were attending.

It became clear after the first visit to School Welfare that some effort to bring the addresses of the children further up to date would cut down the amount of complicated detection work necessary. In tracing the next three groups (41 children born in October and November 1969, 37 children born in December 1969 and January 1970, and 50 children born in February, March, and April 1970), the first port of call was the Grampian Health Board's Community Health Division. Here the organizing secretary was given access to a card index system which recorded, in alphabetical order, all the children born in the city of Aberdeen in a given year. These cards also recorded the name of the general practitioner with whom the child was registered, and any changes of name or address before the child entered school at age four or five. In most cases it was noted that the child had duly entered school, but not the school attended. Information was not available on all the children, but it was possible to confirm or correct a number of addresses up to the point of school entry in 1974 or 1975. Medical records on children after they have entered school are filed at the Community Health Division on an alphabetical basis by school rather than by surname. Since it was assumed that many children would have changed their address between school entry and the beginning of the follow-up study, and that the school they were attending was therefore uncertain, no attempt was made to follow them through any further at this department. Instead, the organizing secretary returned to the School Welfare Department, with the new list of addresses, rearranged on a geographical basis.

Complicated searches were still required at the Department, because the assumption that many children would have moved since starting school proved correct. It seemed desirable to revise the list of addresses still further, and this eventually led to another major modification in the tracing system. By December 1979, a number of telephone enquiries about families who were proving difficult to find had been made to the Grampian Health Board's Primary Care Department, and some useful information had been received. Consequently, in January 1980, the organizing secretary wrote to the Primary Care Administrator to find out about records system maintained by his department, and as a result was given a most instructive guided tour by a member of his staff.

The Primary Care Department's Registration section is responsible for a nominal index of all patients registered with general practitioners in the Grampian Health Board area. The index is organized alphabetically in two sections, one for males and one for females. Knowledge of an individual's Christian names, surname, and date of birth are necessary in order to make use of it. It does not contain any medical information, being simply an index of the names and addresses of patients, and the name of the doctors with whom they are registered. Changes of name and status and of address are constantly being recorded in the index as such information becomes available.

It was clear that this nominal index would provide a relatively up-to-date address for many of the remaining children in the sample, and so in March 1980 the organizing secretary asked the Primary Care Administrator for direct access to it, and subsequently made three tracing visits to the index. At this time it was still a manually operated system, consisting of filing cabinets filled with index cards, so that looking up a group of 50 children involved a full morning's work. The information available from the nominal index proved most useful, though the system was not infallible. If a child did not appear in the index, the chances were either that he had left the area or that there had been some change in family circumstances and that his surname was now different. Frequently, such a change of name could not be tracked down by any cross-references. To keep the index up to date, the records staff were dependent on a flow of information from general practitioners. The quality of this might vary, but general practitioners can only pass on information about changes of address and of name and status if patients inform them and many families do not keep their doctors abreast of such changes.

Accurate information was often not available about families who were in the habit of moving frequently, or who were in particularly unstable domestic circumstances. It was possible to come away from Primary Care Registration with inaccurate addresses and out of date addresses; children might be missing from the index though they were subsequently found to be in the area, or present in the index though they were subsequently found to have left the area. Children or mothers might appear in the index under names they no longer used, and no cross-reference led to the new married or 'also known as' names. Such inaccurate information often created extra difficulties in the tracing process, though occasionally it provided a useful clue along the way.

On the whole, however, the nominal index proved most useful and made it possible to bring a large number of addresses up to date. The index also had the double advantage that, unlike the other systems used, it covered the whole of the Grampian Health Board area and that, once a child had been defined as a tracing problem, it could be used to institute a search for one or other parent, which sometimes made it possible to find a child who did not appear in the index.

After a tracing session at the Primary Care Registration section, it was necessary to organize the information gained on a geographical basis, and then go on to the School Welfare Department to seek final confirmation of the addresses, and check on which schools the children were attending. At the end of each such session, a number of children remained who appeared to be living in the residential areas on the outskirts of the Aberdeen District which were not covered by the School Welfare Department records. To confirm the whereabouts of these children, who numbered 45 in the whole study, telephone calls were made to the appropriate primary schools. Many such calls were also made in relation to children who, according to the records at the Primary Care Registration section, were living elsewhere in the Grampian Region.

A total of 224 of the 296 children were thus traced by way of searches carried out at the School Welfare Department, at the Community Health Division followed up by a visit to School Welfare, or at the Primary Care Registration section followed up by a visit to School Welfare. This figure includes those about whom confirmatory telephone calls had to be made to the schools.

THE TRACING PROBLEMS

A total of 72 children proved impossible to find by way of the basic tracing methods, and therefore came to be categorized as tracing problems. These were children known or believed to be living elsewhere in Scotland, in England or abroad, or children who because of family mobility or changes in name due to alterations in family circumstances had either fallen out of the various records systems or were impossible to locate within them because of insufficient information. Such children might in fact still be living in the Grampian Region, and could prove just as difficult to find as children who had moved elsewhere. One child who constituted a major tracing problem, for instance, was eventually found to be living at the address in Aberdeen at which his parents were resident when he was born; it was still officially the family home, though they had been absent from it and resident elsewhere for long periods, and certainly were not living there when the tracing began. Thus, even when there was evidence to suggest that a child had left the Aberdeen area, it was useful to start by counter-checking at the Primary Care Registration section and at the School Welfare Department. Much time could be wasted following up clues that a child was living elsewhere in Scotland or in England, only to find that the move had been temporary and that the family had returned to the area.

Although numerous different methods had to be used to trace the problem cases, the organizing secretary came to use two sources of information as the basis of the search for the majority of them. Her first recourse was to the interviews conducted with the mothers soon after the birth of each baby. These were read through carefully, and every scrap of potentially useful information about the child, the parents, and the family background was noted. From them it was possible to discover the mother's Christian name, and the full name of the father, the father's occupation, and the mother's former occupation. They indicated whether the parents had close relatives in Aberdeen, and how often they were in the habit of seeing them. The names and addresses of married sisters or sisters-in-law living in Aberdeen were recorded, if the mother had any. In two instances this piece of information led directly to a child being traced. As it happened, 20 of the tracing problems (8 LBW and 12 control children) were in the intensive sample, and second interview schedules were also available; no additional information was available from these, unless the mother mentioned some intention of leaving the Aberdeen area.

From the records available at the Aberdeen Maternity Hospital, it was possible to extract useful details, notably the dates of birth of both parents and the mother's maiden name. The Maternity Hospital records give a cross-reference to subsequent pregnancies, and this on occasion would lead to a more recent address than any which had been found, or would indicate a change in married name. One child was traced as a direct result of the latter information. The records also state the address to which the mother and baby had been discharged, and this could provide a clue, especially in association with the mother's maiden name. Two children were traced as the result of a successful search through the telephone directory for a maternal grandmother still resident at the discharge address.

With the majority of the children in the LBW Study sample, who were not difficult to locate, the investigations in the records systems were concentrated specifically on the child. But once a child had been defined as a tracing problem, the search broadened out and the aim became to find either the child, or one or other of this parents, or any relative who might be able to say where the child was living. This was why the organizing secretary initially spent a good deal of time gathering every available piece of information about the whole family. This often meant that several possible lines of enquiry opened up, all or any of which might lead eventually to the child. Sometimes much painstaking and fruitless work was expended on one line of enquiry, and then the child was found relatively easily in another way. Information about parents or relatives gathered from the Study interviews or from the Aberdeen Maternity Hospital records, if appropriate, was followed up at Primary Care Registration and at School Welfare, either by telephone or as part of a tracing session for another group of children.

It was to some extent a matter of chance or convenience which line of inquiry was tried first in any given case. At times, what seemed initially to be the easiest or more obvious line to pursue proved one to abandon, because it might have led to embarrassment or might have been counter-productive. For example, contacting the second spouse of a divorced husband or wife was generally avoided. Equally, if a mother and child had left home because of a history of domestic assault, it seemed undesirable to contact the father for information, even if it was known where he was living.

Useful as educational and medical records were in locating the majority of the children in the LBW Study, establishing a personal link of some kind proved to be invaluable when it came to finding the more elusive cases (Table 6.4). The staff of schools and the relatives of the children concerned were particularly useful contacts. If it was possible to establish that a child had attended a given primary school at any point in his life, the school records or the personal recollections of the headteacher or secretary (based often on an intimate and

Table 6.4   Mechanism by which child presenting tracing problems was finally located

Mechanism	No. of children
Enquiries to schools/local education offices in and out of Grampian	16
Enquiries to families in and out of Grampian	12
Grampian Health Board Primary Care Registration (before used as a routine procedure)	11
School Welfare Department in Grampian	5
Telephone directories	5
Professional directories/enquiries to father's past or present employer	5
School Health Service in Grampian	3
Social Work Department in Grampian	3
Primary Care Registration section or equivalent outside Grampian	3
Aberdeen Maternity Hospital Records	1
Enquiries to hospital outside Grampian	1
Electoral Registration Office—abroad	1
Tracing problems: Total traced	66
Untraced	6
Grand Total	72

lengthy knowledge of the area and the school population) might provide information, such as what school a child had transferred to, what area he had gone to, or what change in family circumstances had accompanied or precipitated a move. Twice comparable information was obtained from a member of staff at a divisional education office.

One child, for example, had lived at many addresses in the Grampian Region. A telephone call to the primary school in a certain village confirmed that he was not in attendance there, but the headteacher offered to consult parents who happened to be in the school at the time, one of whom thought the family had gone abroad. The organizing secretary subsequently wrote to the headteacher, giving some information about the family and about the LBW Study, and asking for further assistance. The headteacher pursued enquiries, and within a few days was able to send a current address and a photograph of the child, supplied by a relative living in the village. Another child who had moved frequently within the Grampian Region was finally found to have attended a certain school the previous year, and the headteacher told the organizing secretary what area he thought the child had moved to. After telephone calls to six schools had drawn a blank, the organizing secretary telephoned the divisional education office, where a member of staff remembered seeing the name on a list of children for whom transport was provided between home and school. A search through the relevant lists yielded the child's home address and the school attended, and it was then possible to confirm the child's whereabouts (and the fact that his address had changed yet again) by a telephone call to the school.

A number of families who had left the Aberdeen area, and some who had not, were eventually found as a result of making contact with a relative. Where telephone calls were made to schools or to families every effort was made to describe the nature of the Aberdeen LBW Study, and to explain precisely why the research workers wished to locate the child. It was stressed that the primary interest was in the child, and that his parents were only wanted in their parental capacity, rather than in any personal capacity. For the sake of speed, the telephone was used whenever possible, but when speaking to a school secretary, a headteacher or a relative, the organizing secretary always offered to put her explanation about the LBW Study and her request for information into writing if they preferred it.

It was only rarely that anybody asked how their address, telephone number or connection with a child had been discovered. Two mothers and two aunts did ask how they had been located, and a precise explanation was given. The organizing secretary also offered such an explanation voluntarily on several occasions, if there was reason to think she was speaking to a middle-aged or elderly relative who might be made anxious by unexpected enquiries about members of the family. Several times, a string of clues led to the telephone number of a child's parents, rather than the address, and in such instances a direct telephone call was made asking them for their address and the name of the school their child attended. Such calls were always followed up by the usual correspondence.

Tracing the problem cases would have been infinitely more difficult without frequent recourse to the telephone which, although time-consuming, was still quicker and more likely to elicit information than writing letters and awaiting replies to them. Numerous letters were written, however, to relatives, schools, education offices, professional bodies, consular offices, and one electoral registration office. Such letters contained detailed information about the Aberdeen LBW Study, and why it was wished to establish contact with a particular family.

When children were living or thought to be living outside the Grampian Region, one of the difficulties posed by the effort to trace them was that all possible sources of information had to be located. The addresses and telephone numbers of education offices, schools, Primary Care Registration sections or their equivalents, employers, relevant professional bodies, and so on all had to be found, and this added to the overall tracing problem.

Telephone directories were heavily used to elicit information of this kind, as well as information relating to particular tracing problems. Much time was spent trying to locate individuals or possible employers through Directory Enquiries, and perusing telephone directories with the same end in view. A number of visits were made to the General Post Office in Aberdeen to consult directories. On one occasion an outdated Glasgow area directory was used to confirm that an address known to be incorrect in 1980 had still been correct in

1977. Contact was then made with the primary school which the child was most likely to have been attending in 1977, and this school was able to provide a forwarding address, which in turn had to be confirmed with the appropriate school. Information about the movements of a child's father was provided on several occasions by a telephone call to a past employer. Contact with area health board Primary Care Registration sections or their equivalents outside the Grampian Region was always made by telephone (numbers were available from *The Hospitals and Health Services Year Book* and from telephone directories and enquiries made by telephone). As often as not, this source of information was used to confirm that a family had left a particular area, but on several occasions useful clues about the movements of a family were obtained. The address of one child was located as the result of a call to the Primary Care Registration section covering that part of England from which his father was known to have come before settling in Aberdeen.

The telephone directory covering Aberdeen and North-East Scotland was a useful source of information, once the first names of a child's parents were known. The efficacy of directory searches to find or confirm addresses was somewhat hampered for several months, however, because as a result of industrial action the 1980 directory for the area was delayed, and addresses in the 1978 directory, the latest available, could not be relied on. During this period, Directory Enquiries were also unable to provide the numbers of new subscribers or numbers which had changed when subscribers had moved.

When a child's parents or a known relative had a very common surname, it would have been possible but was in fact totally impracticable to make telephone calls to everybody of that name in the appropriate directory in the hope of locating them. On a number of occasions when a relatively unusual name was involved, however, the organizing secretary did work through a whole list of names, having first drawn up a list of priorities based on her knowledge of family circumstances and the geography of the Aberdeen District and the Grampian Region and on a certain degree of intuition. Two of the children living abroad were located because their mothers had rather unusual maiden names, and their maternal grandmothers were found by way of a directory search followed by a number of telephone calls. One such search designed to find a paternal grandparent led directly to a child's parents, who had returned to the Aberdeen area after a number of years.

Telephone enquiries of this kind proved taxing and were potentially embarrassing, whether they drew a blank or were successful. When a family proved difficult to trace, a bereavement, a separation or a divorce was often at the root of the problem. (Of the 32 LBW and 20 control children known to have been affected by such events, 13 LBW and 12 control children were among the 72 tracing problems.) Sometimes these events had already come to light, sometimes they had not, but in any situation it was necessary to tread delicately when making enquiries of relatives. The approach was always to offer a full explanation about the Aberdeen LBW Study, and to stress that the primary interest was in locating the child. In the course of telephone enquiries, contact was made with five aunts, an uncle, seven grandmothers, a cousin, and one divorced parent. On two occasions, the whereabouts of a child was finally discovered from the second spouse of a divorced parent. Several letters were sent to relatives asking for information but none produced a response. Telephone enquiries were sometimes greeted with understandable caution initially but, once the necessary explanations had been made, the recipients were always remarkably courteous and, on those occasions when they were in fact related to a child, helpful as well. Only one family appeared to be deliberately evasive.

Grandmothers, when they could be found, were a most reliable source of family information, regardless of whether a child's original family unit had proved stable or not. Even when families had split up, grandmothers (unlike some other relatives), appeared to maintain at least a friendly interest in their grandchildren, and knew who they were living with and where they were living, either precisely or in general terms which provided useful clues. On one occasion, for example, the paternal grandmother did not know the new married name of the child's mother, but knew what area they were living in, and provided the names of the child's older and younger siblings. Armed with this information, it was relatively easy to find the child's new surname and address through a telephone call to the appropriate school.

COMMENTARY ON TRACING THE SAMPLE

In addition to the original LBW Study register and the interview schedules conducted with the mothers, 24 different sources of information were used to trace the ten-year-old children for the follow-up study. They were:

    School Welfare Department—Grampian Regional Council
    Social Work Department—Grampian Regional Council
    Community Health Division—Grampian Health Board
    Primary Care Registration section—Grampian Health Board
    School Health Service—Grampian Health Board
    Aberdeen Maternity Hospital records
    Royal Aberdeen Children's Hospital records
    Enquiries to other hospital departments, or to hospitals outside Aberdeen
    General practitioners/health centres
    Divisional education offices in Grampian Region
    Headteachers and secretaries of primary schools—in Grampian Region and elsewhere
    Enquiries to relatives
    Directory Enquiries

Telephone directories
Enquiries to father's last known place of employment
Directories relating to father's employment—General Medical Directory, university staff list, etc.
Enquiries to organizations relating to mother's profession—General Teaching Council, General Nursing Council, etc.
Newspaper clippings relating to families in Study
Visits to last known family address
Random personal knowledge of members of staff or colleagues
Education offices outside Grampian Region
Primary Care Registration sections or equivalents outside Grampian
Emigration/consular offices
Electoral registration office—abroad

The high success rate in tracing the sample, and the high proportion of the children still living in the Grampian Region, often at addresses unchanged since their birth or since 1974, both conceal the difficulties that were in fact experienced (Table 6.5). Even addresses which proved to be correct had to be confirmed and tracing the children who came into the problem category was complex and time-consuming. Many of the families still living in the Grampian Region had moved in and out of it during the decade, and some had lived at numerous addresses within it. Of the 32 LBW and 40 control children who constituted tracing problems, 20 LBW and 23 controls eventually proved to be living within the Region. The address at which a child was eventually located was not necessarily an indicator of how easy or how difficult it had been to find him (Table 6.6). Outline case histories of certain of the children who proved most difficult to locate will give an indication of how complex an operation it was.

One child still appeared in the Primary Care Registration nominal index at the address in the register used as the baseline for the follow-up, but according to the records at the School Welfare Department he was not living there, and the appropriate primary school had no knowledge of him. A different address was obtained for the father from Primary Care Registration, but he did not appear in the telephone directory and Directory Enquiries were not able to supply a telephone number. The appropriate primary school for this address did not know the child. A letter was sent to the father but produced no response. It was known that the parents probably had relatives in Aberdeen, but it proved impossible to locate them. A further search at Primary Care Registration revealed that the father had in fact re-married, and when a new telephone directory came out, a telephone number was found. A call to the second wife provided the child's mother's new married name, and gave an indication of the area they were living in. The precise address was then obtained by enquiries to several schools.

Table 6.5   Home addresses at original study and follow-up

	LBW	Control
Original address still correct	35	37
New address recorded before mid-October 1974 still correct	35	28
Address changed	78	83
Total	148	148

Table 6.6   Location of sample

	LBW	Control	Total
Aberdeen District	122	116	238*
Rest of Grampian Region	14	16	30
Rest of Scotland	5[1]	6[1]	11[2]
England	3	3[1]	6[1]
Abroad	2	3	5
Untraced	2	4	6
Total	148	148	296

* Includes 3 children whose parents refused permission for them to take part.
( ) Children interviewed at Institute of Medical Sociology while on holiday in Aberdeen

The mother of another child had indicated at interview when the child was ten months old that the family would soon be moving to England. A check with Primary Care Registration confirmed that the family was no longer in the area and no relatives could be located. No trace of the family could be found in the records of the appropriate Primary Care Registration section in England. Enquiries to professional bodies with which the parents might have been registered in England and Scotland drew a blank, while the personnel department of the organization which had employed the father stated that he was no longer in their employ. It was subsequently deduced that the father was likely to have worked at a certain branch of the organization after his move to England, and the personnel department there eventually discovered that he had died. The rest of the family were thought to have 'gone back North'. Enquiries were then made to the Primary Care Registration section in the area in which the mother's parents were known to have lived, and these resulted in an address dating back several years. The local authority education offices were contacted to find out what school the child was likely to be attending if the address were correct. A member of staff at the education officer took up the search and was eventually able to provide the mother's new married name, a new address and the name of the school the child was attending.

In the case of a third child, two different sources of information indicated that the family had moved abroad, but no address was known. Primary Care Registration confirmed that the family was no longer in the Grampian Region. It seemed probable that one set of grandparents might be in Aberdeen, but efforts to trace them through hospital records and by a visit to one known address proved fruitless. The other grandparents were known to be deceased, and efforts to trace one known relative met with no success. The emigration office through which the family would have passed had no records about them, because they had left Britain too long ago, but the staff there advised which consular office to contact. This office in turn provided the address of the electoral registration office in the state in Australia to which the family was thought to have gone. A letter was sent to this office, which in due course provided an address for the family. This proved to be correct, and contact was established with them.

INTERVIEW PROCEDURES

The success of the field work in a research study depends not only on locating as many of the subjects as possible but also on the degree of their co-operation once they have been found. This in turn may be influenced by the approach made to them by the research workers. In this study the response rate was extremely high, and we are much indebted to both the parents and the children for their co-operation. In all, 282 of the 296 children were interviewed in 1979 – 80. Of the 14 children who were not seen, 6 were untraced and 5 were living abroad, while in 3 cases co-operation was refused.

It was originally decided to conduct the medical examination and the intelligence tests for the follow-up study in the childrens' schools, principally on the grounds that they were likely to feel less apprehensive and to perform better in a known environment. Interviewing at school also meant that parents would not be subjected to any inconvenience, and therefore might be more likely to co-operate. The accuracy of this expectation was confirmed by an early deviation from the original plan.

The first few children were interviewed in July 1979, just before the schools closed for six weeks' summer holidays. In order to keep the interviewing to schedule, it was decided to see 12 children at the outpatients department of the Royal Aberdeen Children's Hospital during the holidays. Seven children were successfully interviewed, but it rapidly became clear that this arrangement was administratively complex, and subject to delays and, more significantly, that parents had to expend much time and trouble to arrange for their child to attend the hospital for what amounted to a two and a half to three-hour session. The families who came to hospital were offered reimbursement for travelling expenses, but not all would accept.

The five children who had not been able to attend for interview at the hospital were subsequently seen at school without any difficulty. It was then agreed that the interview programme should be concentrated in the schools, as had originally been intended, and that the programme should be compressed at the beginning and the end of each school term, in order to include children due to be seen during the school holidays. Interviewing the children at school involved the medical officer and the psychologist in a considerable amount of travelling, but it had the advantage of reducing the demands made on parents.

From late August 1979, the usual procedure was that parents were sent an explanatory letter about the LBW Study, reminding them of their earlier participation and asking for their further co-operation. This was accompanied by a permission form and a stamped addressed envelope for its return. They were told that the medical examination and the intelligence test would take place at school, but that it would not be necessary for them to be present. They were invited to contact the LBW office if they wished for further information or explanations. Eight parents made further enquiries by telephone, usually about the nature of the medical examination, before giving permission for a child to take part.

A number of children were in the care of the local authority and, in cases where the authority had assumed parental rights, permission for the child to take part was obtained from the social worker responsible for him, an explanatory letter being sent to his foster parents.

If there was no response to the first letter after a reasonable period of time, the parents were contacted by telephone if possible. This often meant telephoning out of office hours. Quite often parents had simply omitted to return the permission form, and would either send it back the next day or give permission verbally. Sometimes a parent was doubtful about whether to allow a child to take part and welcomed the opportunity to talk about the Study. On one occasion, the organizing secretary obtained permission from a child, after a lengthy telephone conversation. It was clear that a number of parents allowed the child to make the decision on participation. Very little active hostility was encountered from parents. If the family was not on the telephone, a second letter, not a repeat of the first one, was sent, along with another permission form and another stamped addressed envelope. In most cases, this form was subsequently returned by the parents.

When there was no reason to think that a family would have strong objections to the LBW Study, but it was believed that they were unlikely to send back forms of any description, the assistance of the school was sometimes enlisted. In several instances, an additional permission form handed to the child at school was returned by him to the school, signed by the parent, and then sent on to the Study office. On a few occasions, the medical officer or the psychologist visited families who were not on the telephone to discuss the Study. If parents were simply indifferent, then persuasion was used, but no pressure was put on parents who did not wish their child to take part (Table 6.7). After permission

Table 6.7   Parental response to follow-up study

Response	No. of parents		
	LBW	Control	Total
Permission form returned after first letter	107	116	223
Initial contact with parent made by telephone —verbal permission given	2	1	3
Permission given as result of telephone call following first letter	12	8	20
Permission form returned after second letter	13	9	22
Permission given as result of telephone call following second letter	2	1	3
Permission given after additional letter/ form sent home with child from school	3		3
Permission given after home visit	2	1	3
Permission obtained from social worker	2	3	5
Number of children interviewed	143	139	282
Contact by letter with parents living abroad	2	3	5
Parents refused permission	1	2	3

had been received from parents, a brief letter was subsequently sent with the dates and times of the interviews arranged for their child at school.

Only three parents refused permission, two pleading the extreme nervousness of the child, and the third expressing fears about the nature of the medical examination. In general, the research team's efforts to create as little inconvenience as possible for the parents while at the same time ensuring that they were adequately informed, paid dividends in an excellent parental response. A number of parents contacted the organizing secretary by letter or telephone, asking for a report on their children after they had been examined. In these cases either the medical officer or the psychologist would get in touch with the parent, by telephone if possible (Table 6.8).

Six parents asked to be present at the medical examination at school, and this was arranged. A few parents or children expressed a preference for both examinations to take place at home—apprehension on the part of the child about being singled out from his classmates at school being the most common reason given for this. In four cases the necessary arrangements were made for the medical officer and the psychologist to see the child at home, either during school hours by arrangement with the school, or after school hours. On two occasions, when the interviewer had to travel long distances to see a child, they asked to do so at home because of the difficulty of working within school hours. Three children who lived outside the Grampian Region were brought to the Institute of Medical Sociology by their parents while on holiday in Aberdeen, and interviewed there. Apart from these children, and the seven seen at

Table 6.8   Additional contact with parents

Reason for contact	LBW	Control	Total
Special arrangements for interviews	7	7	14
Parents phoned requesting additional information before giving permission	4	4	8
Parents requested post-interview report on child from doctor or psychologist	10	2	12
Parent wished to attend medical examination at school	3	2	5
Parent at hand (a) At Royal Aberdeen during interview Children's Hospital outpatients dept.	5	2	7
(b) At home	3	3	6
(c) At Institute of Medical Sociology	1	2	3

Table 6.9   Location of interviews

Place	LBW	Control	Total
Schools			
(a) Local authority primary schools	117	126	243
(b) Local authority special schools for mentally/physically handicapped	9	–	9
(c) Private fee-paying schools	5	5	10
Hospitals			
(a) Long-term inpatients	2	–	2
Temporary inpatients	1	1	2
(b) Outpatients	5	2	7
Institute of Medical Sociology	1	2	3
At home	3	3	6
Total	143	139	282

Table 6.10   Number of schools at which interviews took place

Schools	1 pupil	2–7 pupils	8–14 pupils
In Aberdeen District	9	32	11
In remainder of Grampian Region	23	3	–
Beyond Grampian	13	–	–

the outpatients department at the Royal Aberdeen Children's Hospital, and four seen in hospital, all the children were interviewed at school (Table 6.9).

A letter of explanation about the Study, backed up by an additional information sheet, was sent to each school some days before the first pupil was due for interview; precise arrangements about the dates and times of the interview were subsequently made by telephone. Schools were always notified in advance when more of their pupils were due for interview, and then arrangements were made by telephone. As a general principle, the medical officer and the psychologist interviewed a child at school on different days, except in cases where they had to travel some distance to reach the school, when the interviews were usually conducted one after the other. The children who were examined at the Institute of Medical Sociology and the outpatients department at the Royal Aberdeen Children's Hospital were also seen by the medical officer and the psychologist consecutively. The co-operation of school staff was of the utmost importance, and was throughout of the highest order. The Aberdeen LBW Study appeared to create genuine interest in the schools, and this was particularly evident in schools visited by the research workers on a number of occasions (Table 6.10).

TRACING THE SAMPLE IN LONGITUDINAL RESEARCH STUDIES

Tracing the 296 ten-year-old children proved a complex task, which demanded more time and tenacity than had been anticipated in the original research proposal. The 72 tracing problems can be divided into three categories of difficulty (Table 6.11). The first category comprised 26 cases and it took from 1 to 5 steps or procedures to locate these children. Certain of them were found relatively easily early on in the follow-up study, before the Primary Care Registration section records came to be used as a routine procedure, and might not have been classed as tracing problems had they needed to be found later on. There was no real likelihood that this group would not be located. The second category of 35 cases took from 6 to 10 steps or procedures to locate, and the third category of 11 cases from 11 to 17. It is interesting to consider what the effect on the follow-up study would have been, had the 46 children in these two categories not been

Table 6.11   Number of steps taken to locate children presenting tracing problems

| | Steps | | | |
	1−5	6−10	11−17	Total children
LBW	16	13[1]	3[1]	32[2]
Controls	10	22[3]	8[1]	40[4]
Total	26	35[4]	11[2]	72[6]

( ) Child/children untraced.

Table 6.12   Tracing problems: children and pairs

| | Children | | | |
	LBW	Control	All	Pairs
Total	16	30	46	41
Not traced	2	4	6	6
Living abroad	2	3	5	4
Remaining Problems	12	23*	35	31

* Includes 1 child matched with a LBW living abroad,
  and 3 matched with LBW children who were also
  tracing problems

located. Undoubtedly, various kinds of imbalance would have resulted, particularly given that the Aberdeen LBW Study was a case-control study, and failure to find these cases would have made it necessary to exclude their partners also from the results.

An analysis of the 46 tracing problems shows that the group consisted of 16 LBW and 30 control children; 5 of these LBW children were in fact matched with controls from the problem group, so that 41 pairs of children were involved (Table 6.12). Six of the children (2 LBW and 4 control) were not traced and six pairs of children eventually had to be excluded from the results for this reason. Five of the children (2 LBW and 3 control) proved to be living abroad and were not interviewed, though contact was made with their families and all are known to be healthy children, free from handicap, and attending normal schools. Two of these children constituted a matched pair, so a further four pairs had to be excluded on the grounds of geographical location. Ten pairs of children were thus excluded from the follow-up study because one or other or both of them could not be traced or could not be interviewed.

There thus remained 35 children (12 LBW and 23 control) who were classed as tracing problems, but were eventually located and interviewed. One of the control children was paired with a LBW child living abroad, and 3 were paired with LBW children who were also in the problem category, so had none of the 35 been found it would have resulted in the loss of a further 31 pairs. Table 6.13 shows that in addition to the 6.7 per cent of pairs who had to be excluded, a further 20.9 per cent of pairs would have been excluded if the rest of the tracing problems had not been found. This would have meant that in all more than one-third of the children who weighed 2000 g or less at birth, and more than two-fifths of the children whose fathers were in non-manual occupations when they were born, would have been omitted from the follow-up study. Even as it is, the follow-up study is biased in favour of heavier babies and those born to manual workers.

Table 6.13   Effects if tracing problem pairs had been excluded (sample: 148 pairs)

		Not traced or living abroad $n = 10$	Tracing problems $n = 31$	Total $n = 41$	Sample
Pairs	%	6.7	20.9	27.6	148
LBW $\leqslant$ 2000g	%	13.0	23.9	36.9	46
LBW $>$ 2000g	%	3.9	19.6	23.5	102
Boys	%	6.8	23.3	30.1	73
Girls	%	6.7	18.7	25.4	75
Social Class					
Non-manual	%	11.4	31.4	42.8	35
Skilled manual	%	5.9	13.7	19.6	51
Other manual	%	4.8	21.0	25.8	62

The geographical scatter of the tracing problems is interesting to note. Of the LBW children, 5 were eventually found to be living in Aberdeen, 4 elsewhere in the Grampian Region, 2 elsewhere in Scotland and 1 in England; by contrast, 9 of their control partners lived in Aberdeen, 2 elsewhere in Grampian and 1 elsewhere in Scotland. (Of the 3 children among these who were also tracing problems, 1 lived in Aberdeen, 1 in Grampian and 1 elsewhere in Scotland). Of the control tracing problems, 6 were found to be living in Aberdeen, 6 elsewhere in Grampian, 4 elsewhere in Scotland and 3 in England, whereas their LBW partners had proved much less mobile, and 17 were living in Aberdeen and 2 elsewhere in Grampian.

It is not surprising to find that social mobility was one of the contributory factors making children difficult to find, and that a number of tracing problems, both LBW and control, were resident somewhere other than the place of their birth. More surprising, given that the children were matched for social class and for ordinal position in the family, is the degree of imbalance between the numbers of LBW and control children who proved to be tracing problems. There were 16 LBW compared to 30 controls, and this relationship was confirmed by the number who were not traced, 2 LBW and 4 control. If this were proved to be other than a random finding, but was confirmed by the results of comparable studies, the implications for longitudinal case-control studies would be serious. Regardless of how accessible the sample group proves, effective follow-up may always be jeopardized if the control group proves markedly more difficult to find. This indicates how seriously the task of re-establishing contact with the subjects of longitudinal research studies must be taken, and highlights the importance of devising effective tracing methods.

The methods used to trace the children in the Aberdeen LBW Study altered with experience and increasing expertise, but the possibility remains that more efficient ones may have existed. There were undoubtedly records systems and sources of information which might have proved useful, but to which little or no recourse was made. No use was made of electoral registers, for example, principally because it was children who were the subject of the study, and the bulk of the tracing concentrated on locating the children. If adults had been the subject, or if a decision had been made to concentrate on finding the parents of the children, electoral registers would probably have been used. Only minimal use was made for tracing purposes of the records available at the Royal Aberdeen Children's Hospital, although these records were methodically examined by the Study's medical officer after the children had been interviewed and assessed. If certain information about the families had been readily available at the beginning of the follow-up, the organizing secretary's approach to the tracing might have been modified (more use could have been made of telephone directories for example, if the Christian names of the fathers had been known). If it had been realized sooner how much use the nominal index at the Primary Care Registration section would be, this would certainly have been used as a routine tracing mechanism from the start. A system of trial and error is inevitable, however, when methods have to be devised from scratch.

The particular nature of the problems in any specific longitudinal study depend on the personal characteristics and geographical spread of the sample, the records systems to which access is available, and the overall responsiveness to sociological and/or medical research in the area in which the research is being conducted. It is probable, for example, that many local authorities do not have a system similar to that operated by the School Welfare Department in Aberdeen, and it is undoubtedly true that the population of Aberdeen is remarkably well attuned and responsive to field research studies.

Things change rapidly, however, and even a matter of months after the completion of the field work for the Study, the basic procedures which were found so valuable in tracing the majority of the children, may no longer be so effective. Transfer to computer of the nominal index of patients maintained at the Primary Care Registration section will inevitably affect the way in which it can be used. Though a computerized system may be easier to keep accurate and up to date, it may also eliminate the kind of record searching that yields the occasional unexpected but useful clue about family relationships. When it comes to detection work, a drawer full of index cards which have to be painstakingly gone through by hand has its virtues. A computerized system may also be less accessible to a research worker who is not trained to use it, in which case more demand must be made on other people's time than was made in the course of the field work for the Aberdeen LBW Study.

Similarly, the unique and admirable system operated by the School Welfare Department in Aberdeen was altered even before the completion of the field work. The school welfare officers, their current books about their areas, and their collection of retrospective records, were removed to new premises, while the Chief School Welfare Officers and his clerical staff, whose wealth of accumulated knowledge gave such a remarkable added dimension to the operation of the school welfare service, were detached from them and removed to the Grampian Regional Council's headquarters elsewhere in Aberdeen. In the last weeks of the field work for the LBW Study, after these moves had taken place, the organizing secretary had a query about a child. Previously, it would have been resolved by two brief telephone calls in the space of about 15 minutes; on this occasion she had to go to the office in which the books were being stored and seek out the information herself, a round trip of one and a half hours from her own office and back.

Such rapid changes in the records systems in a particular area of Britain suggest that it would be most difficult to build up any useful core of information for the use of research workers engaged in comparable studies in the same area, let alone anywhere else. On the other hand, from the experience gained it is clear that success in tracing the subjects of any similar follow-up study would be facilitated if certain basic family data were gathered together at the outset, and stored in one filing system in one location. For a study involving children, who are likely to be easier to trace than adults as long as the co-operation of the education authority can be secured, appropriate data would be:

The full name and date of birth of the child
The full names and dates of birth of any siblings
The full names and dates of birth of both parents
The mother's maiden name, and previous married name or 'also known as' name (if any)
The address at which the family is resident and their telephone number
The full names, dates of birth, addresses, and telephone numbers of both the maternal and the paternal grandparents

The date of birth is a critical piece of information, and the use of medical records systems, such as the nominal index at the Primary Care Department's Registration section, is virtually impossible without it. Though people may change their surnames and their marital status, their date of birth is permanent. In an area such as north-east Scotland, where certain surnames are extremely common and certain Christian names are not only traditionally popular but may be used repeatedly in different generations of the same family, the date of birth may be the only distinguishing feature which makes the positive identification of a particular individual possible. Telephone numbers should also be recorded as a matter of course if a follow-up study is anticipated within a few years. Of the 290 families traced for the Aberdeen LBW Study, only 49 (26 LBW and 23 control) were not on the telephone, but it was only possible to ascertain this after they had been traced.

In a period when family units are increasingly subject to change, and when the names by which women and children are known are quite likely to alter after a few years, the problems of maintaining or re-establishing contact with the subjects of longitudinal research studies are likely to increase rather than decrease. In view of this, there is much to be said for establishing a coherent body of information and advice about the records systems and tracing methods which are likely to be of assistance to research workers about to embark on the task of tracing a sample after the passage of some years. Teele and his colleagues considered this whole area in an interesting paper on 'Sample Maintenance and Ethical Issues in a Longitudinal Research Study', presented at the 1978 Meetings of the American Sociological Association in San Francisco. He detailed the procedures used by his own research team, and argued that: 'We need more researchers who will tell us about the difficulties in locating respondents in longitudinal studies'. In this chapter, we have attempted to make our contribution to fulfilling this need.

Chapter 7

The Follow-Up Study: Psychological Aspects

C. FRASER

REVIEW OF THE LITERATURE

Results of previous studies

In assessing the intellectual status of low birth weight (LBW) children, account must be taken of variations in the definition and composition of the LBW samples to be considered. Over the years, there has been a change in the composition of the LBW population due, in the main, to improved medical practice. More infants of very low birth weight (VLBW) are now surviving and are believed to be especially susceptible to impairment. Thus, in comparison with earlier studies, a greater proportion of the LBW population as a whole will comprise these VLBW infants. Techniques of medical management have varied not only over time but also from one centre to another and, unfortunately, not all have been advantageous to the infant, e.g. the early starvation regimen employed in the early 1950s.

Research workers have used differing upper weight limits in constructing LBW samples. While many have used 2500 g (5½lb) as recommended by official bodies such as the World Health Organization and the Committee on Hygiene of the League of Nations, others favoured 1500 g or even 1000 g. In general, the earlier studies considered infants weighing 2500 g or less while

Note In the tables and figures in this chapter, degrees of statistical significance are indicated as follows:-

    * = significant at 0.10 level
   ** = significant at 0.05 level
  *** = significant at 0.02 level
 **** = significant at 0.01 level

those in the 1960s tended to use 1500 g as the upper limit or 2500 g in combination with gestational age categories. This changing practice in part reflects growing interest in the ever increasing number of VLBW infants who survive and partly the relatively favourable outcome reported in follow-up studies of heavier infants weighing 2000 – 2500 g at birth.

The terms 'low birth weight' and 'prematurity' were used interchangeably in much of the earlier literature, the implication being that LBW infants are also of low gestational age. More recent studies have noted the importance of gestational age in relation to birth weight, differentiating between the light-for-dates or small-for-dates infant, whose birth weight is significantly below the mean for his gestational age, and the truly premature or pre-term infant, whose low birth weight is appropriate for his shorter length of gestation. In the former group, fetal growth has been retarded, while in the latter, growth has proceeded at a normal rate but the infants have been born before the end of the normal period of gestation. It has been found that these two groups differ not only in the reasons for low birth weight but also in the degree of intellectual impairment. These important differences are obscured in studies which only use the criterion of birth weight when selecting LBW samples.

In assessing the influence of LBW on subsequent intelligence, it is essential to consider the effects of socio-economic status, which correlates significantly with birth weight and, independently of this relationship, with intelligence. Therefore, studies of the influence of LBW on intellectual ability may in fact be studies of the effects of socio-economic status, unless there are appropriate controls. Most of the studies to be considered have employed controls with varying degrees of success, but differing socio-economic distributions between them makes comparison of results difficult. While some do not give precise information on the sample distribution (e.g. Lubchenco et al., 1963), those that do may use samples with a distribution reflecting that of the general population (e.g. Drillien, 1964; Rubin et al., 1973), with a predominance of infants of low socio-economic status (e.g. Eaves et al., 1970) or with many from the non-manual classes (e.g. Dann et al., 1958).

The main features and findings of studies on LBW children over the last thirty years are presented in Tables 7.1 to 7.3. Table 7.1 includes those studies which used LBW samples of 2500 g (5½lb) and less; Table 7.2 those with samples of 2000 gm (4 – 4½lb) and less; and Table 7.3 those with samples of 1500 gm (3lb) and less. In each table, the studies are presented in chronological order with respect to the subjects' dates of birth.

The majority of infants from the studies in Table 7.1 weighed above 2000 g (4½lb) at birth. Thus in the study by Douglas (1956), only 8.8 per cent weighed less than 4lb; in the Baltimore Study (Knobloch et al., 1956), 71 per cent weighed between 2000 and 2500 g; in the study by Rubin et al. (1973), 80 per cent weighed 2000 to 2500 g; and in Drillien's study (1964), 74 per cent weighed above

4 lb. Each of these studies on 'heavy' LBW samples reported that the children were impaired to some degree in terms of IQ scores, school achievement, and incidence of mental subnormality in comparison with a control group. However, the authors had varying degrees of success in matching the controls to the LBW infants for variables such as socio-economic status. Thus Drillien (1964) had an excess of non-manual controls, while Neligan and his colleagues (1976) had a deficit of non-manual prematures and an excess of manual prematures. Douglas (1960), in a revaluation of his sample at 11 years of age, found disparities in favour of his controls in terms of father's employment and of mother's care of the child and interest in school progress. He concluded that the LBW children were no longer significantly impaired, attributing their poorer performance to their inferior family background. However, amongst those pairs considered at that time to be correctly matched, handicap was still evident in the LBW subjects, although of lesser degree than previously postulated. Furthermore, Douglas showed that when the environment favoured a LBW child relative to a control, the former tended to do better than the latter but not to a significant degree, whereas when the environment favoured the control, the LBW child was significantly disadvantaged. Thus parental circumstances do not entirely account for the discrepancy between the two groups. Robinson and Robinson's LBW infants (1965) comprised a group involved in a special neonatal programme along with an equal number not involved in the programme but matched for the same variables as the controls. In order to analyse the effects of birth weight, Robinson and Robinson combined these two LBW groups and compared all infants who weighed less than 1500 g with those weighing 1500 – 2500 g and with the controls. This rearrangement produced, in the smallest weight group, an excess of families of lower socio-economic status as well as an excess of less educated mothers. De Hirsch et al. (1966) failed to match IQ scores adequately, while mothers of their LBW group tended to be better educated. Only two studies, those of Rubin and colleagues (1973) and of the Baltimore group (Knobloch et al., 1956; Harper et al., 1959), expressed satisfaction with their matching. In most cases, the disparities mentioned favour the controls, so diminishing what at first seemed the major role of birth weight itself in causing the relative impairment found. Without further analysis, it is thus difficult to assess the amount of impairment which can be attributed to a low birth weight. Robinson and Robinson (1965), the Baltimore group (Wiener et al., 1965, 1968), and Neligan and colleagues (1976) each employed statistical techniques to eliminate the effects of any mismatching from their analysis. Both Neligan and the Baltimore group found that their LBW infants remained relatively impaired. Robinson and Robinson noted that the impairment of their LBW groups disappeared and concluded that their data did not indicate that LBW children fared any less well than control groups on a variety of intellectual and behavioural assessments.

Table 7.1 Studies using low birth weight samples of 5½ lb or 2500 g and less

RESEARCHER(S)	ORIGINAL SAMPLE	FOLLOW-UP SAMPLE	TESTS EMPLOYED	MAJOR FINDINGS
Douglas (1956) UK	From National Maternity Survey 1946. All legitimate singletons. 675 LBW; 675 FBW matched for sex, ordinal position, mother's age, social group, degree of crowding in home and, where possible, same local authority	Subnormals excluded. At 8 years, 60.4%	Unspecified tests of mechanical reading, word comprehension, and picture intelligence	LBW showed slight but significant impairment in all 3 tests, greatest handicap found in reading
Douglas (1960) UK		At 11 years, 52.6%	Unspecified mixed verbal and non-verbal intelligence tests, reading, vocabulary, arithmetic tests, 11 + results, teachers' comments	1. LBW significantly worse in all tests 2. 9.7% LBW and 22% FBW gained Grammar School places 3. Teachers made more adverse comments about LBW (31%) than FBW (20%) re attitudes to work, discipline and concentration
Robinson and Robinson (1965) USA	All born 1948 – 51. 282LBW; 141 FBW matched for race, sex, birthplace, father's occupation, mother's marital status, parity, attendant at birth, and whether infant was result of single/multiple birth. See text for further details	Major physically handicapped excluded. At 8 – 10 years, approx. 54%	S-B, Goodenough, Jastak Wide Range Achievement Test (reading), Grade Placements, Teachers' Behavioural Ratings	No significant differences in IQ scores reading ability, behavioural ratings and grade placements when social background factors controlled by convariance analysis
Knobloch et al. (1956) USA	The Baltimore Study All singletons born 1952. 585 LBW; 585 FBW matched for race, season of birth, parity, hospital of birth and socio-economic status	Subnormals included. At 40 weeks, 84.8%	Gesell	1. % above average intellectual potential; LBW below 1500 gm 5.3%; LBW 1500 – 2500gm 16.3%; FBW 21.8% 2. % with some neurological and/or intellectual handicap; LBW below 1500 gm 50.9%; LBW 1500 – 2500 gm 28.7%; FBW 12.8%.

Study	Sample	Tests	Findings
Wiener et al. (1965) USA	Subnormals excluded. At 6–7 years, 67.9%	S–B. Goodenough, Bender, Lincoln Oseretsky, rated for speech maturity and 'thinking mode'	1. FBW did significantly better in all except Goodenough. Bender and 'thinking mode' most significant. 2. On removing index of neurological damage from analysis, the significant relationship between LBW and IQ disappeared
Wiener et al. (1968)	Subnormals excluded. At 8–10 years 70.2%	WISC, Bender, WRAT (reading and spelling) rated for speech articulation and complexity of grammar	1. All scores showed increasing impairment with decreasing birthweight 26% LBW and 13% FBW had IQs 50–79 2. WISC better indicator of LBW than Bender 3. Significant differences greatly reduced when effect of neurological impairment removed
Wiener (1968)	Those at special schools excluded. At 12–13 years 72.6%	Used results of most recent reading, arithmetic and intelligence tests given at school, and grade placements	1. 45% of smallest LBW, 57% heavier LBW and 72% FBW in correct grades 2. Birthweight significantly related to achievement, especially in arithmetic tests 3. On removing effects of neurological impairments, birthweight still a significant correlate of academic achievement

Table 7.1 cont'd

RESEARCHER(S)	ORIGINAL SAMPLE	FOLLOW-UP SAMPLE	TESTS EMPLOYED	MAJOR FINDINGS
Drillien (1964) UK	595 infants born 1953 – 55. Twins included, 2/3 LBW; 1/3 FBW selected by being next birth of mature infant after every alternate LBW birth	Subnormals included At 6 months – 7 years At 5 years, 85%	Gesell, Griffith, S – B, Moray House Picture Test, BSAG	1. LBW increasingly impaired as birthweight declines 2. Mean IQ scores: FBW 108, LBW 4½ – 5½lbs 103, LBW below 4½lb 92. 3. Excess of dull and retarded in LBW. Out of 35, 1 was FBW and 1/3 b≥low 3lb 4. Mean score on BSAG increased with decreasing birth weight. Main problems were lack of concentration and feelings of insecurity
De Hirsch et al (1966) USA	Selected in retrospect from larger surveys. Excluded subnormals and those with IQ scores ± 1 Standard deviation from 100. All born 1955 – 56. 53 LBW; 53 FBW with similar background as LBW in terms of mother's employment, attendance at kindergarten and number of times read to. Tested kindergarten to Grade II level		Bender, Oral Language, Reading, Writing and Spelling Tests	1. LBW showed poorer performance on all tests 2. Evidence that rate of LBW progress greater than for FBW 3. Considering only those with IQ scores 90 – 105, LBW performed less well with only Bender and reading tests in Grade II still statistically significant
Rubin et al (1973) USA	Born 1963 – 64. 78 LBW, 32 with GA of 37 weeks or less and 46 with GA of more than 37 weeks; 163 FBW, 78 with GA of 37 weeks or less and 85 with GA of more than 37 weeks	At birth to 7 years At school age, approx. 90%	Bayley, S – B, ITPA, WISC, WRAT, grade placements and problems at school	1. On all measures, FBW did significantly better 2. No significant differences between gestation groups 3. LBW showed consistent impairment in all academic areas 4. Significant higher incidence of neurological abnormality in LBW group

Study	Sample	Tests	Findings
Neligan et al (1976) UK	From Newcastle Survey of Child Development. All singletons born 1961–62. Subnormals included and sample selected in retrospect from main survey. 200 LBW, 141 light for dates (GA of more than 36 weeks and below 10th centile) 59 prematures (GA of less than 37 weeks and below 90th centile). Light for dates divided into rather light for dates (RLFD) 10th-5th centile and very light for dates (VLFD) below 5th centile. 187 FBW. A random sample with similar socio-economic distribution as main survey	Major tests were ITPA, WPPSI, Frostig Pegboard, Skemp Test of Visual Motor Concepts, Bender, Lincoln-Oseretsky, report on behaviour from mother, teacher and psychiatrist	1. WPPSI: Prems and VLFD significantly worse than FBW 2. ITPA: Mean score of LBW differed significantly from FBW but was reduced between 5 and 7 years, suggesting LBW catching up 3. Bender: Very significant impairment between VLFD and FBW and RLFD. Prems performed intermediately, with no significant differences with any other group 4. Neurological impairment found in Prems and especially in VLFD 5. Excess of hyperactive children in Prems and especially in VLFD
Fitzhardinge and Steven (1972) Canada	131 LBW singletons born 1960–66. Only small for dates with GA of 38 weeks and more and at least 30% under expected weight; 36 FBW comprising siblings of same sex and nearest in age to LBW	Subnormals included. At 4–8 years, 73.3% of LBW	S–B, Vineland, WPPSI, WISC, Goodenough, Bender, progress at school	1. For LBW, mean IQ for girls 101 and boys 95. 25% of boys scored below 80. For FBW mean IQ for girls 102 and boys 106 2. 50% of LBW boys and 64% girls progressing satisfactorily at school 3. 1/3 of LBW with IQ of 100+ failing at school 4. 25% of LBW minimally brain damaged

Table 7.2   Studies using low birth weight samples of 4 – 4½ lb or 2,000 g and less

RESEARCHER(S)	ORIGINAL SAMPLE	FOLLOW-UP SAMPLE	TESTS EMPLOYED	MAJOR FINDINGS
Douglas and Gear (1976) UK	From National Maternity Survey 1946. 163 LBW weighed 2000 g or less, 163 FBW details as in Douglas (1956)	Subnormals included. At 15 years, 42%	Watts Vernon reading Test, Graded Arithmetic Test, Alice Hein 4 verbal and non-verbal tests	1. LBW consistently worse on all tests, especially non verbal. None of findings significant. 2. FBW had slight educational advantage in terms of qualifications and higher education entrance
McDonald (1964) UK	1128 LBW born 1951 – 53. Twins included. No controls.	Subnormals included. At 6 – 9 years 94%	S – B	1. Mean IQ for singletons 96.8 or 98.4 corrected for prematurity. 2. 2.7% with IQ below 50 compared to 0.4% in population. 3. Excluding those with major physical defects, mean IQ was 102.4 with an almost normal distribution.
Eaves et al. (1970) Canada	Born 1958 – 1965. 502 LBW, distinguished between SFD and prems; 207 FBW with similar social class distribution as LBW sample.	Subnormals excluded. Infancy 6½ years 67% FBW included only at infancy	Griffiths, S – B, Bender, WISC, Goodenough, Vineland	1. In Infancy, LBW performed significantly less well. 2. No significant differences between SFD and Prems but SFD better in first year while prems did better from 2½ years.

The Baltimore research team (Wiener *et al.*, 1965, 1968; Wiener, 1968) considered that much of their LBW group's intellectual deficit was due to neurological impairment. They combined items from perinatal data and from neurological examination at 40 weeks of age to produce an index of neurological damage: when this was co-varied out of their analysis, the relationship between LBW and intellectual performance diminished and in some instances disappeared. Evidence that neurological factors are involved in much of the impairment found was also provided by Rubin and colleagues (1973), who noted a significantly higher incidence of neurological abnormality in their LBW group; by Fitzhardinge and Steven (1972), who found a higher incidence of minimal brain damage in their LBW group; and by Neligan *et al.* (1976), who concluded that neurological impairment was especially prevalent in their light-for-dates group.

Impairment in school achievement was found in terms of grade placement by Wiener (1968) and of entrance to Grammar School by Douglas (1960). Rubin's group (1973) noted equal impairment in all academic areas examined, while Wiener (1968) found the greatest deficit in arithmetic ability. De Hirsch *et al.* (1966) attempted to equate for IQ scores in their LBW and control groups by considering only those with IQ scores in the range of 90 – 105 but still found that their LBW sample did less well on tests of academic achievement than the controls of similar intellectual potential. Douglas (1960), Drillien (1964), and Neligan and colleagues (1976) also noted an excess of behavioural problems at school, especially in terms of lack of concentration and hyperactivity.

Each of these studies found an excess of major physical and/or mental handicap in their LBW samples. For example, Robinson and Robinson (1965) noted that 24 per cent of their smallest weight group were physically handicapped compared with only 3 per cent of the heavier LBW group and 2 per cent of the controls; Douglas (1956) excluded 11 LBW infants and 5 controls from his analysis due to mental and/or physical subnormality; Wiener's group (1965) excluded, on a similar basis, 46 LBW and 17 control children; and Drillien (1964) found that out of 35 cases of mental retardation, only 1 was a control case.

The findings of the studies in Table 7.2 reinforce the results of the 'heavier' samples in terms of incidence of gross abnormality. However, McDonald (1964) concluded that, if gross abnormality was excluded, her LBW sample did not differ significantly from the test norms. This finding contrasts with some studies in Table 7.1 which excluded the mentally subnormal, such as the Baltimore study and to some extent that of Douglas, which found that significant differences existed. Impairment of the LBW group in comparison with the controls was only investigated by Eaves and colleagues (1970) during infancy: it would have been valuable if they had assessed relative performance up to 6½ years, especially since their was no significant correlation between Griffiths' scores at 6 months and Stanford Binet IQ scores at 4 years, even in children at

Table 7.3 Studies using low birth weight samples of 3 lb or 1500 g and less

RESEARCHER(S)	ORIGINAL SAMPLE	FOLLOW-UP SAMPLE	TESTS EMPLOYED	MAJOR FINDINGS
Dann et al. (1958) USA	116 LBW born 1940–52. Weighed 1000 g or less at birth or during neonatal period. 34 FBW siblings (IQ of LBW with siblings similar to those without so FBW compared to whole LBW sample) Multiple births included.	Not explicit, but gross subnormals appear excluded. At approx. 4–10 years 63%	S–B, WISC, Vineland	1. 44% LBW had IQ below 90; 41% 90–109; 15% above 110 9%. FBW had IQ below 90; 53% 90–109; 38% above 110 2. Mean of LBW 94, FBW 107
Lubchenco et al. (1963) USA	94 LBW born 1947–60. No controls Multiple births included.	Subnormals included. At 10 years 67%	WISC	1. 42% had IQ below 90. 2. 57% with IQ if 90+ had some intellectual handicap. 3. 32% were free of physical and mental handicap.
Drillien (1964) UK	112 LBW born 1948–60. No controls. Multiple births included.	Subnormals included. Infancy - approx. 5 years. 81%	Gesell, S–B, Behavioural Ratings	1. 36% likely to be ineducable at normal school. 2. 33% dull and require special help at normal school 3. 9% of those given IQ test had score over 100. 4. 30% no behavioural disturbance—most common problem hyper-activity.
Wright et al. (1972) USA	70 LBW born 1952–56. 70 FBW matched for sex, race, singleton/twin status, type of delivery, parity, date of onset of pregnancy, socioeconomic status.	Subnormals included At 9–11 years 93%	WISC, Halstead Battery of Neuropsychologic tests.	1. FBW better in terms of IQ scores and school performance. 2. 46% LBW and 8% FBW had IQ below 90; 11% LBW and 45% FBW above 110. 3. 34% LBW unable to attend normal school or doing poorly. All FBW at normal school.

Study	Sample	Age at follow-up	Tests	Results
...and Ramsay (1973) Canada	...priate for dates and weighed 1251 g and less. No controls.	4 – 8 years 82%	WPPSI, WISC, Bender, Goodenough, School Performance.	2. ...40% had IQ below 80, 25% below 80. Mean IQ 88 (boys) and 92 (girls). 3. 31% had perception-motor difficulties. 4. 28% minimally brain damaged. 5. 50% progressing satisfactorily at school.
Francis-Williams and Davies (1974) UK	123 LBW born 1961 – 68. No controls. Distinguished between small and appropriate for date. Multiple births included.	Subnormals included. At 4 – 12 years 85%	WPPSI, WISC, Bender, Neale Analysis of Reading ability, Schonell Graded word	1. Distribution and mean IQ score between SFD and AFD significant (92.0 and 99.2). 2. 15% SFD and 2.8% AFD had IQ below 70. 3. 55.5% of those given Bender scored at least one standard deviation below the norm.
UCH Group Rawlings et al. (1971) UK	72 LBW born 1966 – 69. Multiple births included. No controls but compared IQ scores with those of parents	Subnormals included. Infancy - 5 years, 94%	S – B, Vineland	1. 86.7% mentally and physically normal. 2. Similar IQ distribution to parents. 3. Of 19 given IQ tests, only one had IQ of less than 84
Stewart and Reynolds (1974)	98 LBW. As above and others born 1970	At 2 – 7 years, 97%	S – B, Vineland WPPSI	1. 90.5% had no mental handicap. 2. Similar IQ distribution to parents. 3. 92 had IQ above 80; 4.6% below 68. IQ for younger LBW all above 80.
Turcan et al. (1977)	52 LBW born 1966 – 68, from original Rawlings (1971) sample	At 8 years, 96%	WISC	1. Mean IQ is 95 2. 80% performing satisfactorily in normal school 3. LBW less advanced than classmates in terms of school achievement, emotional and perceptual development

extremes of the scale. We cannot assume that the significant differences found in infancy would have continued into childhood.

In conclusion, the studies shown in Tables 7.1 and 7.2 agree that there is an increased incidence of gross abnormality amongst LBW infants. Lower intelligence scores and poorer academic achievement are also frequently found, though most LBW children fall within a normal IQ range. The inclusion of the mentally subnormal can artificially depress the outcome of the LBW samples taken as a whole (Drillien, 1964; Neligan et al., 1976; Fitzhardinge and Steven, 1972). However, of those studies which specifically excluded the grossly mentally subnormal, only that of McDonald (1964) reported no significant impairment. In the other studies (Douglas, 1956, 1960; Robinson and Robinson, 1965; Wiener and his colleagues, 1965, 1968; De Hirsch et al., 1966; Eaves et al., 1970) impairment was found, though this was noted to be partly attributable to lower socio-economic origins by Douglas (1960) and entirely so by Robinson and Robinson (1965).

Results of the studies listed in Table 7.3 have shown less encouraging results. Dann et al. (1958) alone appear to have excluded the grossly mentally subnormal from the analysis. Information on socio-economic origins of the children was not given by Drillien (1964). In neither of these studies were suitable controls employed. Wright's group (1972) state that they did have matched controls; however, the IQ distribution of their controls (45 per cent above 110, 8 per cent in 70 – 90 range, and none below) suggests that this sample was drawn from the non-manual sector of the population, whereas 55.7 per cent of their LBW group were hospital patients. These design weaknesses are overshadowed by the consistent results found in these studies, which all showed severe impairment in terms of IQ scores. Dann and her colleagues (1958), with a predominantly non-manual population, found that 44 per cent of their sample scored less than 90; comparable figures were: for Lubchenco et al. (1963) 42 (66 per cent private patients); for Wright et al. (1972) 46; and for Fitzhardinge and Ramsay (1973) 40 (28 per cent from Social Classes I and II, 42 per cent from Class III, 30 per cent from Classes IV and V). Drillien (1964) found that only 9 per cent of her LBW sample had an IQ score above 100. School achievement and behaviour assessments also revealed deficits. For example, Drillien (1964) found that some 70 per cent of her sample had behavioural abnormalities, the most frequently noted being hyperactivity, while Lubchenco's group (1963) reported that 57 per cent of their sample with IQ scores above 90 exhibited some deficiency in school performance. In recent years, however, a significant improvement has been noted in the outcome for these VLBW infants and this has been attributed to improved standards of medical care. Francis-Williams and Davies (1974) found mean IQ scores of 92 for their small-for-dates group and 99.2 for their appropriate-for-dates group; Stewart and Reynolds (1974) found that 92 per cent of their sample had an IQ score of above 80, while Turcan et al. (1977) reported that this level of achievement was still in evidence in the same sample at 8 years of age. Socio-economic distribution in the former study was 17.5 per cent in Social Classes I and II, 57.5 per cent in Class III and 25 per cent in Classes IV and V, while for the latter study 37 per cent came from Social Classes I and II, 19 per cent from Class III and 44 per cent from IV and V.

Further evidence that modern medical management of the VLBW infant is producing survivors of better quality has been provided by workers at University College Hospital in London. Stewart and Turcan (1977), comparing the UCH sample over time, found that those born in 1970 – 71 did significantly better in terms of IQ scores on the Stanford Binet scale than those born in 1966 – 67 and 1968 – 69 (mean IQ scores for the three groups were 112, 96 and 98 respectively). This evidence of improvement in IQ scores has been accompanied, however, by the finding of a high incidence of perceptuomotor difficulties with associated learning problems. These workers reinforce the findings of many of the studies previously mentioned: that much of the mental impairment found is the result of neurological deficit, as revealed by scores on the Bender Gestalt test and by neurological examination of the children.

Within the LBW population, does impairment increase as a function of decreasing birth weight?

Studies using 1500 g as the upper limit of birth weight have reported less favourable results than those using a majority of 'heavy' LBW infants, suggesting that the risk of impairment increases as birth weight decreases. Some workers have indeed found this to be the case for their own samples.

1 .The Baltimore group (Knobloch et al. 1956; Harper et al., 1959; Wiener et al., 1965, 1968; Weiner, 1968) noticed a significant trend in favour of the heavier infants as regards intellectual potential in all age groups studied, except in that from 3 to 5 years when the trend was not statistically significant.
2 .Drillien (1964) found that the developmental quotients and intelligence scores increased as birth weight increased, for all social grades.
3 .Neligan and colleagues (1976) found that their 'very light-for-dates' group (mean weight 2397 g) consistently showed increased impairment in comparison to their 'rather light-for-dates' group (mean weight 2701 g) and that in some instances these differences were significant.
4 .McDonald (1964) noted a correlation between IQ scores and birth weight in favour of the heavier infants, in both sexes in Social Classes III, IV, and V; in Classes I and II, the trend was apparent only for girls. She added that there was a small though significant difference between those weighing $3 - 3\frac{1}{2}$ lb and those of $3\frac{1}{2} - 4$ lb, but that children of birth weight 3lb or less showed considerable impairment.

5. Eaves and colleagues (1970) found that, up to 18 months, children weighing 1751 – 2041 g at birth obtained significantly better scores than those weighing 1500 g or less. Thereafter, the difference was reduced, but a clear trend remained.
6. Lubchenco and her group (1963) noted that there was a significantly greater incidence of handicap (mental and physical) in those weighing 1200 g or less compared with those weighing 1200 – 1500 g at birth.
7. De Hirsch et al. (1966) found no gradient in performance with ascending birth weight except in reading achievement scores at the end of the first school grade. For four out of five scholastic tests, however, those who weighed 1500 g or less performed at a lower level than the heavier birth weight group.

A number of studies specify that, within their LBW samples, no significant trend was found relating birth weight to IQ score (Wright et al., 1972; Francis-Williams and Davies, 1974; Dann et al., 1958—though their smallest birth weight group did have a greater incidence of major physical defect; Douglas, 1960; and Robinson and Robinson, 1965). The last of these found that their group who weighed less than 1500 g did worse than those above this weight but they attributed this to the difference in socio-economic distribution found between the two groups which favoured the heavier ones. The findings of some studies (Lubchenco et al., 1963; De Hirsch et al., 1966; Eaves et al., 1970) should be viewed with caution, since they do not allow for any variation in socio-economic distribution between their LBW subgroups. This criticism, however, cannot be levelled at the other four studies mentioned, since both the Baltimore group and McDonald made statistical allowance for such variation, Neligan and his co-workers noted no difference in socio-economic distribution between their 'rather light' and 'very light-for-dates' groups, and Drillien found a positive relationship between birth weight and intelligence within each social grade. The majority of studies which found no significant correlation tended to include only subjects under 1500 g (Douglas is the exception) and it may well be difficult to observe a trend in such a narrow range of birth weights. Thus, it may be stated that evidence, though by no means conclusive, is offered by some of the larger studies, using a broad range of birth weights below 2500 g, to support the hypothesis that mental impairment increases with decreasing birth weight and is independent of socio-economic variations.

Is gestational age at birth important in the progress of the LBW infant?

Some of the investigations previously mentioned defined their LBW samples in terms of gestational age as well as weight at birth, recognizing the possibly independent or interacting effect of these variables.

1. Rubin *et al.* (1973) classified their sample into four groups, defining LBW as 2500 g or less and prematurity at birth as 37 weeks or less. The groups were: (a) full birth weight and full term; (b) full birth weight and premature; (c) low birth weight and full term; (d) low birth weight and premature. They found no significant relationship between the different groups and measures of intelligence. In terms of school progress, however, full birth weight children, regardless of gestational age, did equally well, while amongst the LBW group those who were full term had a higher incidence of educational problems than the premature children. These authors concluded that birth weight rather than gestational age is the major correlate of intellectual impairment but that, amongst the LBW group, the small-for-dates infants constitute the higher risk group in terms of impairment of school performance.

2. Neligan and his colleagues (1976) compared the following three groups: (a) full birth weight, weighing over 2500 g at birth; (b) light-for-dates, having a gestational age above 36 weeks and birthweight below the 10th centile on a weight for gestational age graph; (c) true prematures, whose gestational age was below 37 weeks and birthweight was below the 90th centile. They concluded that, when associated variables had been excluded, their 'very light-for-dates' infants were invariably more impaired than their 'true premature' group.

3. Eaves and her colleagues (1970) defined their LBW groups as follows: (a) small-for-dates, weighing less than 4½lb and on or below the 10th centile; (b) prematures, also weighing less than 4½lb but between the 25th and 74th centile. They noted no significant differences between the two groups in terms of test scores but did notice that their small-for-dates group scored higher in the first year, while prematures had the advantage from 2½ years onwards. The incidence of major defect was higher in their small-for-dates group. Out of 14 exclusions, 10 were small-for-dates.

4. Francis-Williams and Davies (1974) classified their LBW infants as follows: (a) small-for-dates, weighing less than 1500 g and below the 10th centile; (b) appropriate-for-dates, weighing below 1500 g and between the 10th and 90th centile. They found no significant correlation between IQ scores and birth weight or gestational age but their small-for-dates group did score significantly worse on IQ tests than the appropriate-for-dates group. Socio-economic distribution for the appropriate-for-dates was similar to that for the whole LBW sample, while there was a deficit from social classes I and II in the small-for-dates group which would have contributed to their relative impairment.

   Other workers who did not specifically categorize their LBW samples by gestational age at the outset have also considered this issue.

5. Douglas (1956) compared those in his LBW group (2500 g and less) who were born at least four weeks early with term LBW infants and found no

significant differences but he did find a consistent tendency for greater handicap to be found among the least premature.

6. Wiener (1970) found no relationship between IQ scores and length of gestation in his LBW group: amongst his controls, those of shorter gestational age had significantly lower scores. One possible explanation for these results, he suggested, was that bleeding in the first trimester had caused inaccuracy in calculating the gestational age.

7. McDonald (1964), using multiple regression analysis, found no significant correlation between IQ score and length of gestation for her LBW group.

8. Wright and his colleagues (1972) also failed to find any significant relationship between gestational age and IQ score.

From these studies, using a variety of definitions of small-for-dates and premature groups, it appears that gestational age *per se* has no significant effect on intellectual performance but that it does have a significant interactional effect with low birth weight. The small-for-dates infant is found to have a greater degree of impairment than the true premature, the former being born at or near term after intra-uterine growth retardation, while development of the latter has proceeded at a normal rate so that weight is appropriate for gestational age.

Is there a significant interaction between birth weight and socio-economic status?

Evidence on this issue appears to be equally weighted on both sides.

1. Comparing his LBW subjects and controls at 8 years of age, Douglas (1956) found that, for both the vocabulary and the picture intelligence tests, the LBW children of non-manual homes performed better than those of manual workers. Only for the picture intelligence test was the difference significant. However, the later report by this author (Douglas, 1960) that there were significant differences between control and LBW groups in terms of fathers' employment and other items suggests that his findings should be viewed with caution.

2. Neligan and his colleagues (1976) noted, in comparing abnormal groups with controls, that the disparity between them in terms of intellectual ability was most significant in Social Classes III and V while in terms of behavioural assessment Classes IV and V showed the widest disparity.

3. Drillien (1964) showed that the differences in DQ scores between birth weight groups was most marked for the lowest social grades while the correlation coefficient for DQ and birth weight was most significant in Social Class IV. From this she concluded that a combination of inferior genetic endowment, poor environment, and restricted opportunity has a more marked effect on development in LBW groups than in mature infants from similar backgrounds.

4. Eaves *et al.* (1970), in comparing their LBW and control children at 18 months, found significant differences in scores on the Griffiths development test in Social Classes II, IV and V. Evidence for any interaction between birth weight and social class was weak, since the children were very young when tested. Moreover, children from both superior (Class I) and average (Class III) environments showed no significant disparity.
5. The Baltimore workers (Wiener *et al.*, 1965, 1968) noted consistently that LBW children of the lower social classes were not relatively more impaired than those from higher classes. The effect of birth weight, they concluded, was uniform for each social class.
6. McDonald (1964) also noted a constant difference in IQ scores between birth weight groups for each social class.

Thus, the suggestion that LBW infants from lower social groups are relatively more impaired than those from high socio-economic groups is still a matter of some debate. The major studies in this field have produced conflicting results, with Neligan and Drillien finding that an interaction does exist while Wiener and McDonald provide evidence to the contrary.

Summary

From the studies considered, a number of conclusions can be reached:

1. 'Heavier' LBW infants, in general, are minimally if at all impaired intellectually.
2. The very low birth weight groups are more severely impaired though recent reports suggest that there has been a significant improvement, attributed to better techniques of care of the LBW infant.
3. There is an excess of mentally retarded children in LBW groups; this was reported in all the studies.
4. Academic achievement of LBW children is impaired, even of those with average or better intelligence.
5. There is evidence from some reports that LBW children tend to be hyperactive and to lack concentration.
6. Neurological deficit or minimal brain dysfunction has been frequently postulated as the reason for the impairment in performance of LBW children.
7. There is some evidence to suggest that, within the LBW group, intellectual impairment is functionally related to birth weight.
8. Gestational age does not seem to have an independent effect on performance but does interact with birth weight in such a manner that the LBW infant born after a relatively long gestational period is more impaired in later life than the LBW infant of shorter gestational age.
9. Evidence is divided on the question of whether socio-economic factors inter-

act with birth weight, causing those from low socio-economic groups to be more impaired than those from superior environments.

SELECTION OF PSYCHOLOGICAL TESTS

The psychological tests employed in our research study were closely matched to its objectives, which were threefold. First, we wished to obtain an evaluation of each child's level of general intellectual ability; second, we were interested in the children's performance at school and any history of remedial education; and third, we wished to identify those children who exhibited signs of minimal brain dysfunction (MBD). There has been much discussion of the syndrome of MBD by neurologists, psychiatrists, paediatricians, and psychologists, with varying definitions being applied, so we must first consider what we mean by the term.

Clements and Peters (1962) defined it as referring to children with near average, average or above average intelligence who manifest certain learning or behavioural disabilities which are associated with minor deviations of function of the central nervous system. These deviations may manifest themselves by various combinations of impairment in perception, conceptualization, language, memory, control of attention, impulse or motor function. As this definition implies, there is no one pattern of signs which a child must exhibit to be considered to have MBD; rather he will manifest a selection of the following: poor motor co-ordination, poor balance, strabismus, poor speech, poor visuomotor co-ordination, specific learning deficits, short attention span, hyperkinesis, distractibility, impulsiveness, confused laterality, perseveration, and emotional lability; he may also exhibit an abnormal EEG pattern. Many studies have emphasized the diverse nature of this syndrome. For example, Paine *et al.* (1968) found seven independent and unrelated symptom clusters. Most of the neurological abnormality could be accounted for by two of these, namely, perceptual deficits and motor inco-ordination. The other clusters comprised abnormal EEG patterns, abnormalities of reflexes, abnormal prenatal history, and, finally, a factor related to birth order and maternal age which these authors said reflected increased fetal risk. Thus, we would expect our LBW group to exhibit many more signs of MBD than our control group. MBD is of concern to many professional disciplines, as will be clear from the range of signs listed, so that elements of both the medical and the psychological examinations must be brought together to create a true picture of a child's disability. In the psychological examination, emphasis was placed on detecting those children with poor visuomotor co-ordination, specific learning deficits, hyperactivity, easy distractibility, impulsiveness, and/or short attention span. Clements and Peters (1962) suggested that some of the following may appear in the psychological records of children with MBD:

1. Spotty or patchy intellectual deficit.

2. Below mental age level on performance of drawings tests.
3. Poor geometric drawings.
4. Poor performance on block design tests.
5. Poor performance on group tests of intelligence, achievement, and reading.
6. A marked scatter within WISC, with a marked disparity between verbal and performance scales in either direction

In conclusion, as Sattler (1974) states, 'an important criterion in the recognition of minimal brain dysfunction is that the child fails to learn despite an adequate intelligence level and that this disability is not due to severe neurological handicap, emotional disturbance or socio-economic disadvantage'.

The first and major part of assessment consists of a test of intelligence. It is important to remember that intelligence is not an object or 'thing'; rather, we infer a person's intelligence from his behaviour, with intelligence tests acting as sampling mechanisms. Numerous activities can be characterized as being indicators of a person's intelligence, so that many definitions of intelligence have been formulated but none has been universally accepted. As Butcher (1968) says:

> If human intelligence is best described as a statistically unitary trait but also as diverse in its manifestations . . . it is natural that attempts to define it have proved very various. In fact, it will probably always be a misguided labour to try to pin down one and only one logically essential feature of such a flexible and superordinate concept.

One approach used in attempting to describe the structure of intelligence has been to employ factor analysis techniques. Charles Spearman was the inventor of this statistical method and by its use he postulated a two-factor theory of intelligence. He stated that the performance of every cognitive task depended on a general intelligence factor (g) and one other factor entirely specific to the particular task. British psychologists led by Burt and later by Vernon modified Spearman's theory to account for correlations found among cognitive tasks when (g) was removed, and suggested a hierarchical model of abilities. They considered (g) to be at the peak of their model, followed by group factors such as a verbal factor which would be common to a large group of tests, and finally a specific factor pertaining to the individual test. American psychologists, led by Thurstone, used a different factor analytic approach and concluded that there was no general factor but rather seven primary factors. These were described as spatial ability, verbal fluency, numerical ability, perceptual speed, verbal meaning, memory, and reasoning ability. Later, however, Thurstone realized that scores on these factors were correlated, implying a second order general factor. Thus Spearman's attempt to make general intelligence the only common element in cognitive performance and Thurstone's attempt to exclude it were both unsuccessful and have led to a coalescing of views. Most theorists, using factor analysis, now agree on the importance of both general and group factors, with the general factor being the integration of 'lower' abilities.

Burt (1955) defined intelligence as an innate general cognitive ability, emphasizing the importance of the genes we inherit in determining the level of our intelligence and maintaining it fairly constant through life. The nature/nurture controversy has persisted for years and many research workers have striven to discover the relative importance of these influences by considering:

1. Children reared in a uniform environment with differing genetic endowment, e.g. children in a foster home.
2. Children with identical genetic endowment but reared in different environments, i.e. identical twins separated at birth.
3. Identical and fraternal twins, assuming that, if the correlation between the two sets is the same, then environment is important while, if the correlations are different, genetic influences are of primary importance.

Conclusions from these studies have shown that the either/or controversy is meaningless and that an interaction of the two variables is a more tenable viewpoint. Undoubtedly, heredity plays an essential part in determining the limits of intellectual development but environmental factors are important in helping the individual to attain these limits. In this respect, Hebb's definition of intelligence is worthy of note. He distinguishes between intelligence A, which is our innate potential—the brain's capacity for development—and intelligence B, which he defines as the functioning of the brain in which development has occurred and which he considers is related more to experience or, in physiological terms, consists of permanent changes in the organization of pathways in the cerebrum via the establishment of cell assemblies. Neither can be observed, he adds, but intelligence B is a much more direct inference from behaviour than intelligence A. Vernon suggested the addition of intelligence C to this model, that is, the level of intelligence which is measured by an intelligence test and is an estimate of intelligence B.

Thus the intelligence we measure is not a 'pure' intelligence but an inferred level which approximates to our 'working' level of intelligence derived from the interaction of heredity and experience. Factor analytic studies have shown that measured intelligence contains a general integrative factor as well as several 'lesser' group factors which pertain to aspects of intellectual ability.

To measure the children's intelligence for the purposes of the present study, an individual test was required in order to observe the subject's work methods, to find out in which areas he had most difficulty and to gain a general impression of his personality and behavioural characteristics, especially those already mentioned with reference to the brain dysfunction syndrome. There are only two major tests of intelligence which have been widely used in the past, the Stanford Binet Intelligence Scale and the Wechsler Intelligence Scale for Children (WISC). Both are considered reliable and valid assessments of children's intelligence. The Stanford Binet (SB) has a reliability coefficient of 0.83–0.93 depending on IQ level and the age of the child tested. Concurrent and predictive validity of the Stanford Binet have been reported mainly in terms of academic achievements as a criterion and most studies in this respect have found correlations between 0.40 and 0.75, the higher correlates being found with such verbally orientated subjects as English and History. The WISC, too, is a reliable instrument with a reported full scale reliability coefficient of 0.92, verbal scale of 0.96, and performance scale of 0.89. There has been criticism about the lack of validity data on the WISC. However, as regards concurrent validity, studies involving a variety of ages and IQ ranges, as reported by Littell (1960), have found that the WISC and Stanford Binet are significantly related; most reports find a correlation in the region of 0.80. Littell also reports that factor analytical studies into the construct validity of the WISC offer support to the distinction between verbal and performance scores.

The main problem with the SB is that there is a preponderance of verbal material and as such it is primarily a measure of scholastic aptitude, penalizing those whose strongest abilities lie along non-verbal lines, those who have language problems, and those from poor cultural backgrounds, a predominance of whom could be found in the LBW population. Indeed, in the WISC standardization sample, children from rural areas and from low socio-economic status homes did better on the performance than on the verbal scale and so would be penalized if given the predominantly verbal SB.

The WISC was well standardized for the Scottish population in 1974, using a random sample of 200 children from each age from 5 to 15 years. The test contains 12 sub-tests grouped into a Verbal Scale (Information, Comprehension, Arithmetic, Similarities, Vocabulary, Digit Span) and a Performance Scale (Picture Completion, Picture Arrangement, Block Design, Object Assembly, Coding, Mazes). The sub-tests are standardized to produce a mean of 10 and a standard deviation of 3 which readily suggests a comparison of ability between tests. Investigators have found, however, that much of this comparison is unjustified. First, extreme care has to be taken in such comparison since the reliability of individual sub-tests varies from 0.5 to 0.8. Newland and Smith (1967) have produced lists of required differences between each combination of sub-tests scores for them to be significant: in general, at age $10\frac{1}{2}$, 4 points are required between sub-tests to be significant at the 0.05 level. Second, as Littell points out, there is a dearth of information on what sub-tests actually measure, most hypotheses appearing to be based on an 'intuitive appraisal of the content'. Factor analysis of the WISC by Cohen (1959) revealed five primary factors. These are:

1. Verbal Comprehension I: a factor which he defined as verbally retained knowledge that is impressed by formal education. This factor is predominantly found in Information, Similarities, and Arithmetic.

2. Verbal Comprehension II: a factor which measures application of judgement following some implicit verbal manipulation. This factor is found mainly in Comprehension and Vocabulary.
3. Perceptual Organization: a factor which is non-verbal and reflects the ability to interpret and/or recognize visually perceived material. This factor is found predominantly in Block Design, Object Assembly, Mazes, and Picture Completion.
4. Freedom from Distractibility: the factor which measures the ability to attend or concentrate. This factor is found in Digit Span.
5. Quasi-Specific Factor: to which no psychological interpretation has been attributed. This factor is found predominantly in Picture Arrangement and Coding.

Thus, it would seem that individual sub-tests are not reliable measures of specific functions but rather are estimates of specific abilities when combined with other sub-tests. As Sattler (1974) says:

'Cognitive acts require complex and multi-faceted behaviour. Reducing the act to a simple category name does not do justice to the psychological processes involved in the task'.

On the basis of factor analysis, Cohen advised against making interpretation for individual sub-test scores and he devised a deviation quotient to compare his factors. Sattler felt sure that in clinical and educational settings, cautious interpretation of sub-test scores may prove of benefit in suggesting hypotheses to pursue further. The original hope of Wechsler that specific patterns of scores would emerge to correlate with specific pathologies has been dismissed by many due to lack of results in tests designed specifically to investigate this. However, studies such as the one by Clements and Peters (1962) of children suspected of MBD have found that many of these children show a wide disparity in scores, doing worst in what would correlate to Cohen's perceptual organization and freedom from distractibility factors as well as between the verbal and performance scale scores (Clements and Peters define disparity between verbal and performance scale scores as $15-40$ points in favour of the verbal scale and $10-30$ points in favour of the performance scale. However, Field (1960) found that, at 10½ years, 23.5 points of difference in either direction are required to be significant at the 5 per cent level). Paine and his colleagues (1968), in their analysis of referred children suspected of MBD, found a greater number than would be expected, using Field's normative data, of children with disparate verbal and performance scales but that the excess was small. They concluded that the increase existed but was not dramatic enough to make it seem all that important. Thus it seems that analyses of scatter of sub-test scores have not proved to be as fruitful as was once hoped. However, such analyses still seem useful in providing tentative hypotheses and to serve as a sign of abnormality, provided the statistical findings of Field and Newland and Smith are adhered to.

One major fault of the WISC is that IQ scores can only be obtained within the range of 45 – 155. The SB has been found to be more accurate for younger subjects and those with extremes of disability. However, since the vast majority of our subjects would be within this range and all subjects were 10 years old, this did not seem a problem for our particular study.

Thus the WISC was chosen for our study since it is a reliable and valid measure of general intelligence for our age group. Separate verbal and performance scales as well as sub-test scores are provided by this test and these can be compared to reveal various strengths and weaknesses in a child's intellectual make-up. Some authors (Clements and Peters, 1962; Paine *et al.*, 1968) have found an increased frequency in verbal/performance scale disparity in groups of children with MBD—in whom we are particularly interested—while Clements and Peters also found that these children did consistently worse in some sub-tests, particularly those which relate to Cohen's perceptual organization and distractibility factors.

A frequent sympton of MBD is poor visuomotor perception and so the children were specifically tested for this, using the Bender Visual Motor Gestalt Test. This consists of nine cards with simple designs drawn on them. The child is instructed to copy each design, with the sample design before him. The designs were selected by Bender to illustrate Gestalten principles of perceptual integration and differentiation. Koppitz (1964) derived a scoring system from a normative study which she carried out on 5 – 10 year olds. By her scoring system, a child should produce fewer errors as he gets older and his visuomotor perception matures, so that by the age of 10 years the average child produces only one or two errors. Koppitz also found that children improve their performance in a fairly standard manner, so that at a specific age certain errors are common while others rarely occur and so are diagnostically significant. She found that children with neurological impairment tend to do poorly regardless of IQ scores and that those who do perform well are likely to have at least average intelligence—they have learned to compensate for their handicap. Thus the Bender Gestalt seemed a useful test to employ in our survey as a measure of perceptuomotor development.

Lastly, we wished to obtain information on the children's progress at school. We wished to find out which children had received remedial education and also which children seemed to be performing at school below their capacity, as defined by their IQ score. It was also considered that it might be useful to gain some impression of the children's behaviour at school, especially to identify those who exhibited behavioural symptoms of brain dysfunction in the classroom. Each teacher, therefore, was asked to fill out a questionnaire. Areas covered included academic performance, history of remedial education, behaviour in class, emotional disposition, incidence of anti-social behaviour, and personality. It is conceded that this may not be the most reliable way of obtaining information, particularly if the teacher has been working for a long time in a particular school where the distribution of children's abilities tends to be skewed, so that the teacher loses touch with what an average 10-year-old is able to do. However, we were only interested in trends of differences between the controls and the LBW group and there seemed to be no reason to suppose that any bias would not be equally distributed between the two groups. The information on remedial education should be accurate and it was felt that the teachers' impressions of the children would be useful when considered along with the psychological and medical assessment of the children.

THE PRESENT STUDY

The focus on this part of our research study is on the psychological assessment of the LBW children at the age of 10 years in relation to their matched controls and on ascertainment of the degree of any intellectual impairment. The analysis will not attempt to indicate the cause of impairment, but will rather describe it and identify, if possible, groups of LBW children most at risk. Many inter-related biological, medical, and environmental factors are known to be associated in the relationship of birth weight to intellectual outcome. In order to allow for these effects and so, first, to reveal the true contribution of LBW *per se* and, second, to ascertain their relative importance in determining the degree of impairment, a multiple regression analysis will be undertaken in Chapter 9. This section of the analysis, then, has two aims:

1. To investigate the nature and degree of impairment sustained by the whole LBW sample.
2. To ascertain whether the actual birth weight below 2500 g, gestational age, sex of the child, and Social Class at birth (as determined by the father's occupation) are important parameters in determining eventual outcome.

THE LBW SAMPLE IN COMPARISON WITH THEIR CONTROLS

Of the 135 matched pairs who were followed up, only four children could not be tested on the WISC due to mental subnormality (an IQ score of less than 50). Two of these children have cerebral palsy, one has epiloia, and one is of extremely short stature. All four of these children were LBW babies. Excluding these four children and their controls, the mean full scale IQ for the LBW sample was 101.52 compared with 105.94 for their controls—a difference which, using the Student's t-test, is significant at 0.02 level ($t = 2.37$; d.f. $= 260$). Less difference was noted in mean verbal IQ score, the respective values for LBW and controls being 100.96 and 104.07; this difference fails to reach conventional statistical significance. The largest and most significant (at 0.01 level) difference was noted in the performance scale, with the LBW sample having a mean of 103.18 and controls 108.17 ($t = 2.808$; d.f. $= 250$). Figure 7.1a shows that the lower mean full IQ score of the LBW group is due to fewer LBW than

Table 7.4 Distribution of IQ scores

Score		Less than 50	50-69	70-79	80-89	90-99	100-109	110-119	120-129	130+	Total
Full IQ	LBW	4	5	5	16	34	28	26	14	3	135
	Control	0	1	5	11	22	38	38	15	5	135
Verbal IQ	LBW	4	6	8	17	25	31	30	10	4	135
	Control	0	2	7	13	23	37	36	16	1	135
Performance IQ	LBW	4	4	1	19	27	35	23	18	4	135
	Control	0	0	4	8	21	45	26	22	9	135

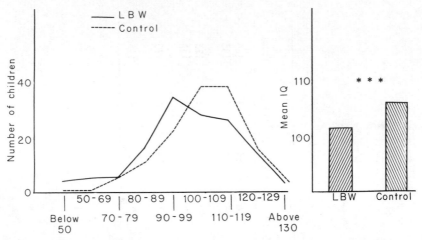

Figure 7.1a   Frequency distribution and mean value of IQ scores: full IQ scale

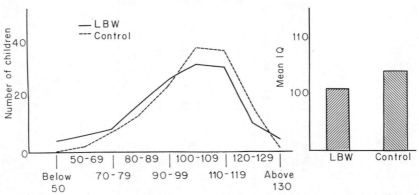

Figure 7.1b   Frequency distribution and mean value of IQ scores: verbal IQ scale

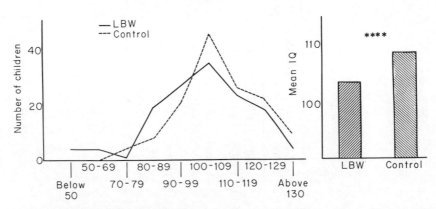

Figure 7.1c   Frequency distribution and mean value of IQ scores: performance IQ scale.

controls scoring average and just above (100 – 119) while more LBW scored below this level. Five LBW children as opposed to 1 control are considered educationally sub-normal, scoring between 50 and 70. At the other extreme of the scale, a similar number of LBW and controls scored well above average (120 and above). Thus, the deficit of the LBW group, in terms of full IQ, appears not to be uniformly distributed across all ranges of intelligence. From Table 7.4 and Figures 7.1b and 7.1c it is apparent that the inferior full IQ scores of the LBW group are due primarily to a deficit in the performance rather than in the verbal scale.

The distribution of scores for the WISC sub-tests (Table 7.5) shows almost uniform impairment in all performance scale tests. In each test, fewer LBW children scored above average (above 12) and more scored below this range. In four out of the six tests (picture completion, picture arrangement, block design, and coding) the difference in distribution was significant at the 0.05 level, using the chi-squared test. While the same trend is apparent for most of the verbal sub-tests, only the difference in distribution for the arithmetic is highly significant (at 0.01 level). These weaknesses in the LBW sample are not contained exclusively in any of Cohen's five groups (see page 153) but pertain mostly to his perceptual organization and quasi-specific factors.

The frequency distribution of scores for the Bender Gestalt test of visuomotor perception (Figure 7.2a) describes the inferior performance of the LBW group with an excess of LBW children scoring five errors or more. Mean score for the LBW group is 3.05 compared with 2.2 for the controls, a highly significant difference at 0.01 level. Koppitz (1964) categorized errors in the Bender test into four types:

1. Distortion errors where the shape of the copied figures have been distorted.
2. Rotation errors where the copied figures have been rotated by at least 45°.
3. Integration errors where there has been a failure to join figures or conversely a joining of them when they should be apart.
4. Perseveration errors where repeated patterns have been inordinately continued.

Figures 7.2b, 7.2c, 7.2d, 7.2e show that the LBW group have made more errors of distortion (mean difference significant at 0.05 level) and integration (mean difference significant at 0.01 level) rather than of rotation or perseveration. According to Koppitz's normative data, mean score at 10 years of age is 1.6 with a standard deviation of 1.67. On this basis, we would expect 50 per cent of 10-year-olds to score 1.6 or less, 83.3 per cent to score 3.27 or less, and 97.5 per cent to score 4.97 or less. From Figure 7.3 we can estimate that 48 per cent of our LBW sample tested on the Bender scored 1.6 or less, 70 per cent scored 3.27 and less and 85.5 per cent scored 4.97 and less. Comparable figures for the control group are 57 per cent, 84 per cent, and 96 per cent, which is a close approximation to the normative data. The LBW group, on the other hand, have an excess scoring more than two standard deviations above the mean.

Table 7.5 Frequency distribution of WISC subtest scores. (a) Verbal scale. (b) Performance scale

(a)

Score	General information LBW	Control	General comprehension LBW	Control	Arithmetic LBW	Control	Similarities LBW	Control	Vocabulary LBW	Control	Digit span LBW	Control
Not testable	4	0	4	0	4	0	4	0	4	0	4	0
Less than 5	16	12	9	2	12	7	2	4	6	2	0	0
5–8	28	23	48	45	30	15	44	33	22	18	44	40
9–11	59	67	33	40	45	71	29	29	52	47	57	55
12–15	25	32	30	38	39	41	49	60	49	67	28	36
Above 15	3	1	8	7	5	1	4	6	1	0	2	4
Total	135	135	132	132	135	135	132	132	134	134	135	135
Sig.	0.191		0.069*		0.002****		0.171		0.063*		0.207	

Note: Some totals are slightly reduced because children were not all tested due to lack of co-operation or lack of time.

(b)

Score	Picture completion LBW	Control	Picture arrangement LBW	Control	Block design LBW	Control	Object assembly LBW	Control	Coding LBW	Control	Mazes LBW	Control
Not testable	4	0	4	0	4	0	4	0	5†	0	5†	0
Less than 5	11	9	2	1	7	3	0	0	3	0	1	1
5–8	60	43	41	28	31	24	17	10	15	16	43	30
9–11	41	60	54	57	57	53	40	40	39	27	54	60
12–15	19	23	32	48	32	46	59	67	54	64	29	38
Above 15	0	0	1	0	4	9	15	18	19	28	3	6
Total	135	135	134	134	135	135	135	135	135	135	135	135
Sig.	0.027**		0.050**		0.050**		0.159		0.025		0.080*	

† Four mentally subnormal children plus one cerebral palsy child who was unable to hold a pencil.

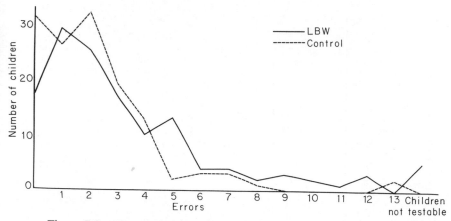

Figure 7.2a   Frequency distribution of Bender scores: Bender score

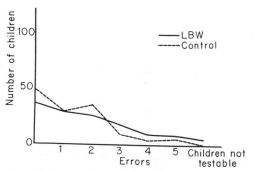

Figure 7.2b   Frequency distribution of Bender scores: distortion

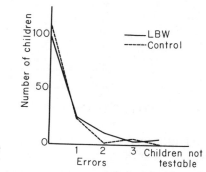

Figure 7.2c   Frequency distribution of Bender scores: rotation

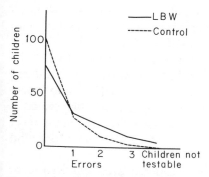

Figure 7.2d   Frequency distribution of Bender scores: integration

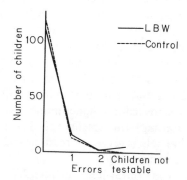

Figure 7.2e   Frequency distribution of Bender scores: perseveration

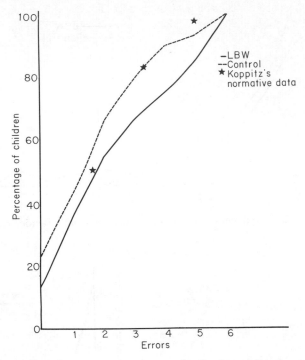

Figure 7.3   Cumulative percentage distribution of Bender scores

Questionnaires were given to the teachers of all children in normal schools and those at the local school for the educationally sub-normal. Excluded from this analysis, however, are the four mentally sub-normal children, two children who were tested in hospital and one cerebral palsy child attending a school for spastics, and their controls. No teacher refused to take part and discrepancies in the total number of recorded scores in Tables 7.6 and 7.7 are due to some teachers missing out certain items. In terms of academic performance (Table 7.6), the teachers rated the LBW sample to be inferior to the controls in all areas, with only the distribution of reading scores for the LBW group failing to be significantly different from the control group. Though more LBW children than controls have received remedial education (37 as opposed to 29) the difference is not statistically significant (probability = 0.317). Thus, although the LBW group tend to have lower IQ scores and to do less well at school, there is not a significantly higher number who have received or are receiving remedial help. Perhaps the reason for this apparently discrepant result is that most remedial help is given for reading and, in this area, the LBW group were found to be least impaired.

On behavioural items (Table 7.7) teachers considered LBW children to be significantly more prone to fidget, to be slap-dash in their attitudes to work, to

Table 7.6   Academic ratings

		Below average	average	Above average	Total	chi-square
Physical	LBW	30	84	13	127	0.002
education	Control	11	92	24	127	****
Essay	LBW	64	44	17	125	0.003
writing	Control	40	51	34	125	****
Spelling	LBW	55	52	21	128	0.0187
	Control	35	59	34	128	***
Arithmetic	LBW	49	48	30	127	0.034
	Control	30	57	40	127	**
Project	LBW	40	63	19	122	0.034
work	Control	23	71	28	122	**
Reading	LBW	42	55	31	128	0.189
	Control	34	50	44	128	
Overall						
school	LBW	46	60	22	128	0.019
performance	Control	32	56	40	128	***

Table 7.7   Behavioural items from teachers' ratings

		Does not apply	Applies somewhat	Definitely applies	Total	chi-square
Fidgets	LBW	58	47	20	125	0.020
	Control	80	31	14	125	***
Slap-dash	LBW	69	42	15	126	0.050
	Control	87	26	13	126	**
Irritable	LBW	105	16	6	127	0.029
	Control	115	12	0	127	**
Frequently	LBW	98	20	8	126	0.039
fights	Control	109	16	1	126	**
Well	LBW	2	37	88	127	0.047
behaved	Control	4	21	102	127	**
Solitary	LBW	73	36	14	123	0.096
	Control	81	37	5	123	*
Anxious	LBW	47	60	17	124	0.071
	Control	65	46	13	124	*
Easily	LBW	49	51	28	128	0.091
distracted	Control	65	45	18	128	*
Concentrates	LBW	21	61	45	127	0.097
	Control	17	48	62	127	*

be more irritable and less well behaved in class and to fight with their peers more frequently than do their control group. Behavioural items which were marginally significant suggested that the LBW children were more solitary, anxious, easily distracted, and lacking in concentration. Most of these differences are suggestive of neurological impairment or developmental delay.

Table 7.8   Clinical impressions of behaviour

		Normal	Doubtful	Abnormal	Total†	chi-square
Impulsiveness	LBW	89	27	17	133	0.002
	Control	113	14	6	133	****
Concentration	LBW	87	23	22	132	0.003
	Control	100	27	5	132	****
Activity	LBW	95	17	21	133	0.013
level	Control	112	14	7	133	***
Personality	LBW	98	22	12	132	0.014
	Control	115	14	3	132	***
Anxiety	LBW	98	21	15	134	0.015
	Control	114	7	13	134	***

		Normal	Doubtful	MBD	More severe	Total	chi-square
Neurological	LBW	67	37	18	13	135	0.003
state	Control	88	31	15	1	135	****

		Normal	Doubtful	Abnormal	Does not speak	Total	chi-square
Speech	LBW	114	12	4	3	133	0.096
	Control	123	5	5	0	133	*

† We were unable to rate all of the mentally subnormal children.

The teachers did not rate the LBW group as different from the controls on many items, including bullying, stealing, and other anti-social behaviour, popularity with peers and shyness. The teachers were also asked to rate the parents' interest in their children's progress. In view of the differences noted in parental attitudes between the LBW and controls in Chapter 4, it was surprising to find that little variation was noted between the two groups. However, more LBW than control parents were reported to show no interest (13 to 5).

Our clinical impression of these children reinforced the behavioural differences noted from the teachers' reports (Table 7.8). We considered the LBW children to be significantly less able to concentrate, to be more impulsive, hyperactive, and anxious, and to exhibit signs of abnormal personality, e.g. excessive shyness, over-confidence, or appearing distant. Our ratings of neurological status, based on the neurological examination, test scores, and clinical impression, revealed that there were similar numbers of LBW and control children who were considered to have minimal brain dysfunction (MBD). More controls were considered to be normal, however, while there was an excess of LBW children showing more severe neurological impairment. This finding is discussed on page 197.

Although the number of LBW children exhibiting a sufficient number of signs to warrant the diagnosis of MBD was similar to the number of controls, the LBW sample as a whole had in psychological terms a greater preponderance of MBD symptoms. The LBW group, from the Bender scores and WISC performance scale, revealed deficit in perceptuomotor skills, had a greater incidence of hyperactive and impulsive children, and contained more children lacking in concentration and showing emotional lability. The number achieving below their potential or showing a wide disparity in verbal and performance IQ scores was similar in the two groups. Although more LBW children were having problems with schoolwork, as shown by poorer academic ratings and the greater number who were receiving or had received remedial help, the difference appears to be commensurate with the greater number of LBW children having IQ scores below average. When comparing the IQ scores of those children receiving or having received remedial help, no difference was noted in distribution, 8 LBW and 7 controls having IQ scores above 100. If more of our LBW children had been achieving below their potential, we would expect the IQ scores of the LBW children who were receiving or had received remedial help to be higher than those of the controls receiving help, and this is not the case. Field (1960), in his normative analysis, found that 11.4 points difference between verbal and performance IQ scores for any child was required to be significant at the 0.05 level and this was noted for 54 LBW and 49 controls. Thus, in psychological terms, the LBW group exhibited a preponderance of many MBD signs but in few children were they of sufficient number or severity to warrant the diagnosis. It has been suggested that, by 10 years of age, many children have learned to compensate for their deficit and it is probable that we have encountered this phenomenon in our sample.

Our results confirm the findings of the majority of previous studies using LBW samples of 2500 g and less. Our LBW group had a greater incidence of mental and educational sub-normality, exhibited impairment on IQ scores, made more distortion and integration errors on the Bender test (which is suggestive of neurological impairment), had lower academic achievement in most areas, and showed a higher incidence of behavioural problems. The Baltimore study is best suited to direct comparison since, although their sample was multiracial, both were case-controlled studies, birth weight distribution is very similar (the Baltimore group had 71 per cent weighing 2001 – 2500 g, 16.5 per cent between 1501 – 2000 g, and 12.5 per cent below 1500 g (Wiener et al., 1965), while our comparable figures are 71 per cent, 22 per cent, and 7 per cent), their subjects were tested at approximately the same age (Wiener et al., 1968), and the same intelligence test was used. In terms of incidences of subnormality and intellectual impairment, our results concur. Wiener noted a difference of 4.9 points in mean IQ between LBW and controls, while our sample showed a

4.4 difference; Wiener had 16 cases of mental or gross physical subnormality out of a total of 433 LBW children (3.7 per cent), while we had 4 cases of mental subnormality in our LBW sample (2.95 per cent); approximately twice as many LBW children as controls had IQs in the range 50 – 79 in the Baltimore study and we noted 10 LBW as opposed to 6 controls. Whereas the Baltimore study noted that most impairment in academic skills was in arithmetic rather than reading or spelling, and Rubin *et al.* (1973) noted a similar degree of impairment in all three, we found that, according to the teachers' reports, spelling, essay writing, and physical education showed most deficit. We agree with the Baltimore group that little impairment was noted in reading. By teachers' reports and/or clinical impression, the LBW group were found to be hyperactive and lacking in concentration and impulse control, which was also noted by Douglas, Drillien, and Neligan. Our group too were considered to be less well behaved and to be prone to fight. In accordance with all studies using the Bender-Gestalt test, significant impairment was found, with errors of integration and distortion being responsible for the deficit. None of the studies of LBW samples using the WISC specifies whether the verbal or performance scale showed most impairment. We noted, however, that deficit in the performance scale was the principal cause of lower full scale IQ score and this is in accordance with the greater incidence of perceptuomotor difficulties noted in our LBW sample.

The low birth weight sample and degree of impairment

Birth weight below 2500 g

In Chapter 5 it was noted that the birth weight of the infant had some influence on the extent of clinical problems in the neonatal period. To find out if the actual birth weight of a LBW infant is important in determining subsequent impairment, a bivariate regression analysis of birth weight on IQ and Bender impairment scores was carried out. The impairment score for a LBW child was calculated by subtracting his score from that of his matched control. Thus an impairment score of 0 means that the LBW child has done equally as well as his control; on IQ scores, a negative score means that he is doing less well and a positive one that he has done better; on the Bender score, the reverse is true, with a positive score meaning an inferior performance. Not all LBW children performed worse than their controls on the WISC and Bender: 38.5 per cent of LBW children had higher full IQ scores than their matched controls while 25.9 per cent of LBW had fewer Bender errors. Figure 7.4, the regression line of birth weight on mental impairment scores, shows that as birth weight decreases, impairment increases. The birth weight at which no full IQ impairment is predicted is 2518 g, suggesting that in terms of IQ deficit, 2500 g is in round figures the correct upper limit of birth weight at which to define children at risk.

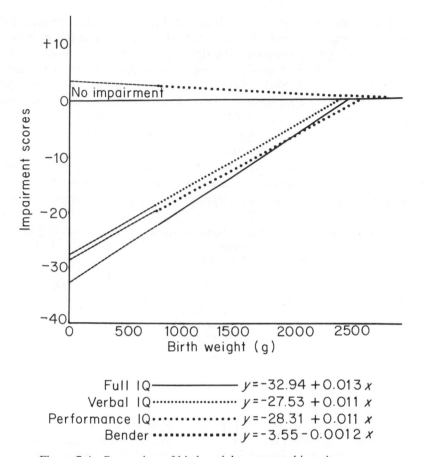

Figure 7.4   Regression of birth weight on mental impairment scores

The regression lines of verbal and performance IQ impairment are similar with no impairment predicted at 2472 g and 2622 g, respectively. Thus a LBW child with a birth weight of 2500 g would be predicted to show no impairment in the verbal scale, while in the performance scale some deficit would be apparent. At lower weights, deficit will be found for both scales, but will be greater in the latter. This is in accordance with the finding of greater impairment noted in performance IQ scores (page 159). Birth weight and full IQ impairment have a correlation coefficient of -0.246 which is significant at 0.01 level. The correlation coefficients for the verbal and performance scales were almost identical with values of -0.207 and -0.198, respectively, and are significant at 0.05 level. In comparison, the regression line of birth weight on Bender impairment (Figure 7.4) predicts no impairment at a higher weight of 2876 g. Thus all LBW children are predicted to show impairment. The correlation coefficient is -0.153 which is not significant and points to a very weak association between birth weight and Bender impairment. Thus most LBW children are impaired on the WISC and Bender test but while actual birth weight is of minimal importance in determining outcome on the Bender test, in terms of IQ impairment, a relationship exists with birth weight, though not a strong one, whereby degree of impairment increases as birth weight decreases. It is important to remember that, at this point, we cannot say that a lower LBW has caused the greatest impairment, but only that lighter LBW children will be more impaired. The regression lines reveal that for heavier LBW children, deficit is minimal in terms of IQ scores but that some impairment is evident in the Bender test. These trends are borne out if we compare the test mean scores for the LBW sample, split into two groups for those above 2000 g and those of 2000 g and less (Table 7.9). In each IQ scale, very significant impairment is noted in the lighter-weight

Table 7.9   Mean impairment scores for birth weight groups (excluding the mentally subnormal)

	Birth weight	
	⩽ 2000 g	> 2000 g
Full IQ	− 11.10****	− 1.77
Verbal IQ	− 9.70****	− 0.51
Performance IQ	− 10.50****	− 2.79
Bender Score	+ 1.33**	+ 0.67*
Integration Errors	+ 0.61****	+ 0.30

group, while children over 2000 g have, on average, sustained minimal impairment especially in the verbal scale. The table of mean Bender impairment again shows that the effect of birth weight is less pronounced, with both groups showing some degree of deficit, though the lighter group again has come off worse. The number of distortion errors was not significantly different for either LBW group in comparison to their controls, whereas the lighter LBW group had significantly (at 0.01 level) more integration errors with no significant impairment noted in the heavier LBW group. Lower LBW appears to be related to a diminution in the integrative function of perceptual skills.

In order to observe any differences in behavioural and academic ratings, the distribution of scores for the same two LBW groups and their controls were compared. There are 97 cases in the group 2000 g and above, with 38 below this weight. This difference in sample size makes comparison in terms of chi-square testing difficult, since similar disparities which appear significant in the larger group may not appear so in the smaller one. This would not mean that the smaller (and in this case lighter) group are any less impaired in our sample but that we are less certain in making inferences about the population of very light babies.

In each academic subject there is a trend in both LBW groups for more LBW than controls to be in the below average category and fewer above average (Table 7.10). In most cases the distribution of control scores is concentrated in the average category, with an even proportion above and below average, whereas for the LBW group the distribution is skewed to the average and below average categories. There is no instance where a group of LBW equal or better their controls. In arithmetic, essay writing, and project work, the disparity between the LBW group less than or equal to 2000 g and their controls is greater than for the heavier LBW group and their controls: this is confirmed by the chi-square test, whereby the disparity is significant in the former group and marginally or not significant in the latter. For reading, neither distribution of LBW scores is significantly different from that of their controls. However, while the distribution betweem the LBW and controls in the heavier group is very similar (29 per cent LBW and 25 per cent controls below average; 41 per cent LBW and 39 per cent controls average; 29 per cent LBW and 35 per cent controls above average), for the lighter LBW group a greater disparity is observed (42 per cent LBW and 30 per cent controls being below average and 11 per cent LBW and 30 per cent controls above average). In spelling, a marginally significant deficit in the heavier LBW group was noted (41 per cent LBW and 25 per cent controls below average, with 58 per cent LBW and 75 per cent controls considered average or better). The lighter LBW group show a similar disparity but due to smaller numbers this difference is not significant (47 per cent LBW and 33 per cent controls below average, 52 per cent LBW and 66 per cent controls average or better). A significant disparity was found in physical education ratings for the heavier LBW group (19 per cent LBW and 7 per cent controls below average, 80 per cent LBW and 93 per cent controls average or better). The lighter LBW group seem to show greater deficit though, again due to the smaller sample size, this is of only marginal statistical significance (33 per cent LBW and 11 per cent controls below average, 66 per cent LBW and 89 per cent controls average or better). The evidence thus tends to suggest that the lighter LBW are more impaired in relation to their controls than are the LBW group over 2000 g, in most academic subjects and especially in arithmetic and essay writing. Only in spelling do the lighter group match the deficit of the heavier. In terms of number of LBW children receiving remedial help, neither LBW group was found to be significantly different from their controls. However, while 23 per cent of controls for both LBW groups had received remedial help, 37 per cent of the lighter LBW and 26 per cent of heavier LBW were similarly rated. It thus appears that the lighter LBW group are showing greater deficit in academic achievement and this is in accordance with their intellectual handicap found in the WISC scores.

On considering those behavioural items from the teachers' ratings which significantly discriminate the whole LBW sample from their controls, there appears to be no consistent trend for the greatest deficit to be found in the

Table 7.10 Academic ratings by birth weight

	Arithmetic				Essay writing				Reading				Project work			
	LBW 740–2000	Cont.	LBW 2001–2500	Cont.	LBW 740–2000	Cont.	LBW 2001–2500	Cont.	LBW 740–2000	Cont.	LBW 2001–2500	Cont.	LBW 740–2000	Cont.	LBW 2001–2500	Cont.
Below average	20† (58)	9 (26)	29 (32)	21 (23)	24 (66)	13 (36)	40 (45)	27 (30)	15 (42)	11 (30)	27 (29)	23 (25)	14 (41)	6 (18)	26 (30)	17 (19)
Average	11 (31)	16 (46)	37 (40)	41 (46)	9 (25)	14 (39)	35 (39)	37 (41)	17 (47)	14 (39)	38 (41)	36 (39)	17 (50)	22 (65)	46 (52)	49 (56)
Above average	4 (11)	10 (29)	26 (28)	30 (33)	3 (8)	9 (25)	14 (15)	25 (28)	4 (11)	11 (30)	27 (29)	33 (35)	3 (9)	6 (18)	16 (18)	22 (25)
Total	35 (100)	35 (100)	92 (100)	92 (100)	36 (100)	36 (100)	89 (100)	89 (100)	36 (100)	36 (100)	92 (100)	92 (100)	34 (100)	34 (100)	88 (100)	88 (100)
chi-square	0.0216 **		0.4125		0.0253 **		0.0584 *		0.1214		0.6145		0.0889 *		0.2316	

	Spelling				Physical education			
	LBW 740–2000	Cont.	LBW 2001–2500	Cont.	LBW 740–2000	Cont.	LBW 2001–2500	Cont.
Below average	17 (47)	12 (33)	38 (41)	23 (25)	12 (33)	4 (11)	18 (19)	7 (7)
Average	17 (47)	16 (44)	35 (38)	43 (47)	21 (58)	25 (69)	63 (69)	67 (74)
Above average	2 (5)	8 (22)	19 (20)	26 (28)	3 (8)	7 (20)	10 (11)	17 (19)
Total	36 (100)	36 (100)	92 (100)	92 (100)	36 (100)	36 (100)	91 (100)	91 (100)
chi-square	0.1058		0.0609 *		0.0511 *		0.0337 **	

Remedial education received

	LBW 740–2000	Cont.	LBW 2001–2500	Cont.
Yes	13 (37)	8 (23)	24 (26)	21 (23)
No	22 (63)	27 (77)	68 (74)	71 (77)
Total	35	35	92	92

† Figures in brackets are percentages.

lighter LBW group (Table 7.11). A definite trend for the lighter LBW to be more impaired was found for only two items. The teachers felt that these children were more solitary and irritable than their matched controls, whereas little difference was found between the heavier LBW group and their controls. The lighter LBW group also showed signs of being more prone to fidget, to be easily distracted, and to lack concentration. No difference between the two groups was noted in terms of abnormal anxiety and the number who frequently fought, while the heavier LBW group were less well behaved and more slap-dash in relation to their controls than the lighter LBW group to theirs. Our behavioural ratings (Table 7.12) show no evidence of an increase in behavioural disorder with decreasing birth weight. The lightest group show a slight excess of anxious children, but with no difference noted in personality disorder and hyperactivity between the two groups. In contrast, the heavier LBW seemed more impulsive and lacking in concentration. Our neurological ratings (Table 7.13), however, do show a birth weight influence, with impairment being more prevalent amongst the lighter LBW, an excess of whom were considered to have MBD or to have sustained more severe impairment.

As birth weight decreases, therefore, there is a trend for greater deficit to be found in intelligence scores, academic achievement, and neurological function. Perceptuomotor skills as measured on Bender impairment scores are found to show little relationship to birth weight but integrative skills are more impaired in the lighter LBW group. Most behavioural abnormalities (including those of possible neurological origin, e.g. impulsiveness, hyperactivity) showed little relationship to birth weight, and in some cases, least deficit was noted in the lighter LBW group. It is interesting to note that, according to clinical impression, more of the lighter LBW children were neurologically impaired and yet the individual psychological components of this rating often failed to show this trend. This suggests that, while individual indicators of neurological impairment are equally prevalent across all ranges of LBW, the incidence of these indicators occurring in combination is greater for the lower ranges of LBW.

Gestational age and low birth weight

One conclusion reached in the literature review was that gestational age had an important interactional effect on birth weight, whereby the LFD infant has a poorer prognosis in terms of intellectual development than the prematurely born AFD infant. However the studies cited have used various definitions of what light-for-dates means. Rubin's group (1973) defined all LBW infants of 37 weeks and over as growth retarded and conversely those of gestational age of less than 37 weeks as appropriate for dates. Neligan and co-workers (1976) used a similar classification to define their LFD group (all infants of 225 days or more and below the 10th centile) and their premature group (all infants of less than 225 days and below the 90th centile). However, this resulted in only three

Table 7.11 Behavioural items from teachers' ratings by birth weight of LBW children. Per cent to whom the behaviour somewhat or definitely applies

Weight of LBW infant	Solitary		Irritable		Fidgets		Distracted		Lacks concentration	
	≤2000	>2000	≤2000	>2000	≤2000	>2000	≤2000	>2000	≤2000	>2000
LBW	50	37	17	17	61	50	66	60	66	63
Control	23	39	3	12	39	35	50	49	50	51
Control − LBW	−27	+2	−14	−5	−22	−15	−16	−11	−15	−12

Weight of LBW infant	Anxious		Fights frequently		Not well behaved		Slap-dash	
	≤2000	>2000	≤2000	>2000	≤2000	>2000	≤2000	>2000
LBW	69	59	20	23	17	36	41	46
Control	55	45	11	14	22	18	28	21
Control − LBW	−14	−14	−9	−9	+5	−18	−13	−23

Table 7.12 Clinical impressions of behaviour. Per cent in whom item rated as doubtful abnormal or abnormal

Weight of LBW infant	Anxious		Personality		Hyperactive		Impulsive		Lacks concentration	
	≤2000	>2000	≤2000	>2000	≤2000	>2000	≤2000	>2000	≤2000	>2000
LBW	26	27	27	25	34	26	31	34	36	33
Control	11	16	13	12	21	13	16	14	13	21
Control − LBW	−15	−11	−14	−13	−13	−13	−15	−20	−5	−12

Table 7.13 Neurological ratings (Percentages in brackets)

	Normal	Doubtful	MBD	More severe	Total	Sig.
LBW ≤ 2000 g	16(41)	10(20)	8(20)	5(13)	39(100)	0.0333
Control	26(27)	9(23)	4(10)	0(0)	39(100)	**
LBW > 2000 g	57(53)	27(28)	10(10)	8(8)	96(100)	0.069
Control	62(66)	22(23)	11(11)	1(1)	96(100)	*

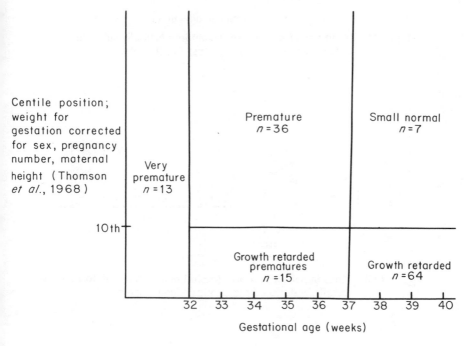

Figure 7.5   LBW sample: centile/gestational age groups

LFD infants who were also premature being included in their premature group. Evidence to be presented here suggests that those children who were both growth retarded and prematurely born are a high risk group. Eaves and her colleagues (1970) and Francis-Williams and Davies (1974) compared all their LBW infants below and above the 10th centile, regardless of gestational age, and so obscured any effect of premature birth.

With these observations in mind, the LBW sample was divided into five groups (see page 95) as shown in Figure 7.5.

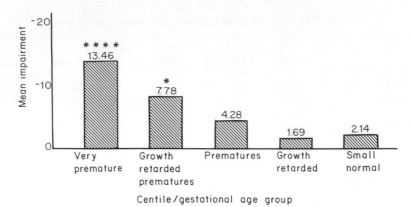

Figure 7.6a   Mean impairment scores (excluding mentally subnormal) by centile/gestational age groups: full IQ score

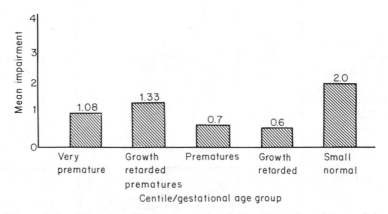

Figure 7.6b   Mean impairment scores (excluding mentally subnormal) by centile/gestational age groups: Bender score

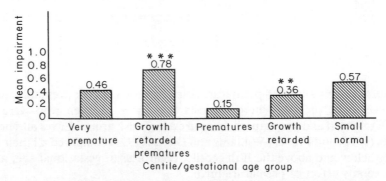

Figure 7.6c   Mean impairment scores (excluding mentally subnormal) by centile/gestational age groups: integration errors

Figure 7.6a shows the mean full scale IQ impairment for each of the five groups. The very premature infants are significantly impaired with a deficit, on average, of 13.46 IQ points. This group, incidentally, had most neonatal problems at birth. The growth retarded prematures show the next greatest deficit which is marginally significant. The premature group are still less impaired, showing the effect of growth retardation in the 32 – 36 week period. No such trend, however, is evident for the LBW groups of 37 weeks and more gestation, with minimal impairment noted in both the small normal and growth retarded groups. Figure 7.6b shows the corresponding impairment for Bender scores, with no group showing statistically significant deficit. Integration errors, again, revealed deficits in specific groups, with all growth-retarded infants showing significant deficit in this test (Figure 7.6c). The very premature group, who showed the greatest impairment in intelligence, do not exhibit any significant deficit on the Bender test. From our neurological assessment (Table 7.14) it appears that severe neurological impairment has not been confined to the most premature or growth-retarded but has been spread across all five of our groups. However, the three premature groups, who also had most neonatal problems at birth, have a deficit of children considered normal.

It is possible that the deficits observed are due, not to particular characteristics of that group, but to differences in birth weight distribution between groups. Perhaps all that is being observed here is that lighter-weight LBW infants are more impaired. Birth weight correlates strongly with gestational age (0.736 in our sample) and so we would expect our more premature

Table 7.14   Neurological ratings by centile/gestational age groups. (Percentages in brackets)

	Normal	Doubtful	MBD	More severe	Total
Very premature	4(31)	5(38)	3(23)	1(8)	13(100)
Controls	12(92)	1(8)	0(0)	0(0)	13(100)
Growth-retarded premature	6(40)	5(33)	2(13)	2(13)	15(100)
Controls	9(60)	5(33)	1(7)	0(0)	15(100)
Prematures	14(39)	11(31)	8(22)	3(8)	36(100)
Controls	22(61)	8(22)	6(17)	0(0)	36(100)
Growth-retarded	38(59)	16(23)	5(8)	6(9)	64(100)
Controls	38(59)	17(27)	8(13)	1(1)	64(100)
Small normals	5(72)	1(14)	0(0)	1(14)	7(100)
Controls	6(86)	0(0)	1(14)	0(0)	7(100)

LBW infants to be lighter and therefore more impaired on IQ scores and integration errors, for example. In terms of average birth weight, our very premature group were much lighter than the others. Mean weights were 1494 g (very premature), 2040 g (growth retarded prematures), 2123 g (prematures), 2303 g (growth retarded), and 2441 g (small normals). In order to determine if any of our observations were due to birth weight distribution, each group was divided into two groups, those above 2000 g and those of 2000 g and less. There were no small normals below 2000 g and only one very premature above 2000 g who was excluded for the purposes of this analysis. Table 7.15 shows that some of the remaining eight groups are very small indeed and it is questionable whether any inference can be made, particularly in lighter birth weight groups.

Table 7.15 Sample size of centile/gestational age groups by birth weight

Weight	Very premature	Growth-retarded premature	Premature	Growth-retarded	Small normal
≤ 2000 g	12	6	14	5	0
> 2000 g	0	9	21	56	7

Figure 7.7a, however, demonstrates a consistent trend for all groups comprising infants of 2000 g and under to exhibit substantial deficit. The very premature group continue to show most impairment but are still lighter, approximately 300 g lighter, than LBW infants in other groups under 2000 g. Therefore, it is suggested that the significant impairment noted in terms of IQ score in the very premature group is due to their very low birth weight. An infant of comparable weight from any group would exhibit similar deficit. Conversely, Figure 7.7a also shows that the heavier groups are minimally impaired apart from the growth-retarded prematures who show a deficit which reaches marginal statistical significance. While for the premature and growth-retarded groups the relationship of lighter birth weight and greater impairment (as found in the section Birth weight below 2500 g, page 166) continues, for the growth-retarded prematures, constant impairment over all birth weights is found. In terms of Bender impairment scores (Figure 7.7b), none of the heavier LBW groups show any significant impairment, with the small normal group, as in the group analysis over all LBW children, showing the greatest deficit. For those LBW of less than 2000 g, significant impairment is noted in the growth-retarded group with the growth-retarded prematures showing the largest deficit but, due to a wide spread of scores, the difference fails to be significant. For all of the heavier LBW groups and most of the lighter LBW groups no significant deficit in integration errors is observed (Figure 7.7c). The growth-retarded group, however,

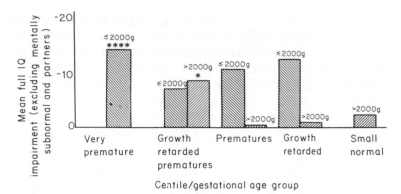

Figure 7.7a   Mean impairment scores by centile/gestational age groups by birth weight: full IQ score

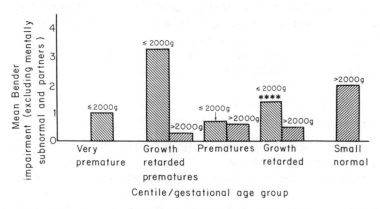

Figure 7.7b   Mean impairment scores by centile/gestational age groups by birth weight: Bender score

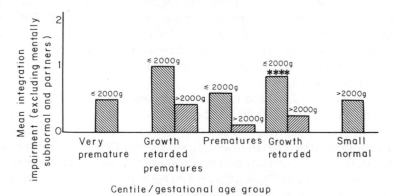

Figure 7.7c   Mean impairment scores by centile/gestational age groups by birth weight: integration errors

are significantly impaired. It seems that the lighter growth-retarded LBW are responsible for the significant integration impairment noted for all growth-retarded LBW, while all growth-retarded prematures are similarly impaired. Due to small sample size, it is not feasible to compare these eight groups on our neurological ratings. It is probable that the deficit in the three premature groups occurred because, on average, these were the lightest babies, and we noted most impairment to occur in LBW of under 2000 g (page 168).

Several observations can be made in relation to these results:

1 .The significant deficit noted in the very premature group has probably occurred because of a preponderance of very light-weight babies.
2 .Evidence suggests that all very low birth weight children (under 2000 g) no matter what gestational age and/or centile position, show signs of intellectual deficit.
3 .For those children above 2000 g, only the growth-retarded premature children show intellectual impairment, with birth weight appearing to have little influence on degree of handicap.
4 .Growth retardation regardless of gestational age appears to result in deficit in the integrative capacity of perceptuomotor skills.

Sex differences and low birth weight

Many research workers (McDonald, 1964; Rubin *et al.*, 1973; Eaves *et al.*, 1970; Fitzhardinge and Ramsay, 1973; Francis-Williams and Davies, 1974) have examined sex differences within their LBW samples, with conflicting results. The reason for this could be that all LBW boys have been compared with all LBW girls and this is fallacious. As Record *et al.* (1969) have shown, at the same gestational age boys on average are heavier than girls and this trend is evident for all gestational ages. Thus, in comparing the sexes, allowance must be made for the fact that in relation to mean weights for all boys, a LBW sample of defined birth weight will include a more 'deviant' sample of boys. The weight for gestational age centile charts compiled by Thomson *et al.* (1968) do make such allowances and so a comparison can be made between the sexes of all LBW children within the same centile range.

Table 7.16 gives mean IQ and Bender impairment scores for all boys and girls on or below the 10th centile and for those above the 10th centile. Those on or below the 10th centile correspond to our growth-retarded and growth-retarded prematures and will be referred to as light for dates (LFD) while those above the 10th centile include the prematures and small normals and will be referred to as appropriate for dates (AFD). Within the LFD group, no significant impairment was observed between the boys and their controls or the girls and their controls for any IQ score, though the boys did now slightly more deficit. In terms of

Table 7.16   Mean impairment scores by sex (excluding mentally subnormal LBW and controls)

Score	Sex	LFD	AFD
Full IQ	Boys	−4.2	−2.6
Impairment	Girls	−2.4	−6.7
Verbal IQ	Boys	−3.7	−2.5
Impairment	Girls	−0.7	−3.7
Performance	Boys	−4.1	−1.8
IQ Impairment	Girls	−3.5	−8.8*
Bender	Boys	1.2****	1.4*
Impairment	Girls	0.3	1.0
Integration error	Boys	0.64****	0.40
Impairment	Girls	0.26	0.25

Table 7.17   Neurological ratings by sex. (Percentages in brackets)

	LFD				AFD			
	Boys	Controls	Girls	Controls	Boys	Controls	Girls	Controls
Normal	24(61)	26(67)	19(51)	18(49)	9(43)	12(57)	10(48)	17(81)
Doubtful	6(16)	10(26)	13(35)	2(32)	5(24)	5(24)	6(29)	3(14)
MBD	6(16)	3(8)	1(3)	6(16)	5(24)	4(19)	3(14)	1(5)
More Severe	3(8)	0(0)	4(11)	1(3)	2(10)	0(0)	2(9)	0(0)
Total	39	39	37	37	21	21	21	21
chi-square	0.166		0.007****		0.468		0.223	

Bender scores, however, the boys showed significant deficit with an excess of integration errors. In contrast, the girls showed minimal impairment. Our neurological ratings (Table 7.17) also suggest that the LFD boys are more impaired (though a more significant disparity was found between LFD girls and their controls due to an excess of LFD with a doubtful rating), with 24 per cent of LFD boys and 8 per cent of their controls considered to have MBD or more severe neurological abnormality, while for the girls the controls had slightly more abnormality than the LBW with 14 per cent LFD girls and 19 per cent of their controls considered to show similar neurological abnormality. Thus, although intellectual ability is minimally impaired for both LFD boys and LFD girls, evidence of greater neurological deficit in the boys has been found, A similar comparison for AFD boys and girls reveals no clear trend, with the girls showing more deficit in IQ scores, particularly for the performance scale (significant at 0.10 level), and the boys showing more deficit on full Bender scores (also significant at 0.10 level). From neurological ratings, more AFD boys than girls showed abnormality but since this also applied to the controls, similar non-significant disparity for both AFD groups in comparison to their controls was found. Thirty-four per cent of AFD boys compared with 19 per cent of their controls and 23 per cent of AFD girls compared with 5 per cent of their controls were rated as having MBD or more severe abnormality.

Our AFD group comprises prematures and small normal LBW children and so it is not surprising that for both boys and girls impairment has not been extensive. However, our LFD group comprises growth-retarded and growth-retarded prematures and so deficit especially in integration errors would be anticipated. This was found to occur but only for the boys, suggesting that the male fetus is especially susceptible to the deleterious effects of growth retardation.

Social class and low birth weight

Of the issues discussed in the literature review, most controversy occurred over whether environmental factors, as measured by father's occupation, have any influence on the degree of impairment sustained by LBW children. While the Baltimore group and McDonald found equal impairment in all social classes, Neligan and Drillien found those of lower social class origins to be more impaired. To investigate the presence of such a trend, the LBW sample was divided into three groups using the criterion of father's occupation at the birth of the child. Thus all children from homes of non-manual fathers (Social Classes I – IIIa) were in one group, those from skilled manual homes (IIIb and IIIc) in another, and those from unskilled manual homes (IV and V) in a third.

Figures 7.8a, 7.8b, and 7.8c show the main test scores for these three LBW groups and their controls. As would be anticipated, for both the LBW and the control group, mean IQ scores decrease as social factors (as measured by father's occupation) deteriorate and this trend is greatest for the verbal rather than the less environmentally influenced performance scale. For each of the three IQ scores, the difference between the LBW and controls is greater for the manual than for the non-manual groups. Mean full scale IQ score for the LBW of Classes I – IIIa is virtually identical to that of their controls (113.4 and 113.9, respectively). In Classes IIIb and c, a six-point and statistically significant (at 0.05) difference is observed (102.6 for LBW and 108.6 for their controls), while in Classes IV and V a similar and marginally significant difference is apparent (94.6 for LBW and 100.1 for controls). It is interesting to note that even with significant impairment, a LBW child from a skilled manual family will, on average, still have a higher IQ score than a control child from an unskilled family, suggesting that a disadvantaged environment will outweigh the disadvantage of LBW. No significant differences are noted in any social group for verbal IQ scores, though once again no impairment is found in the non-manual classes with a 4.3 and 4.0 point difference noted in Classes IIIb and c and in IV and V, respectively. As was found in the whole LBW versus control group comparison, greatest deficit occurs in the performance scale and applies to all social groups. LBW children from Classes I – IIIa show a non-significant 1 point deficit while in Classes IIIb and c and Classes IV and V, significant deficit (at 0.05 level) of 6.3 and 6.6 points, respectively, are noted. In terms of intellectual handicap, then, LBW children from non-manual homes are, on average, unimpaired while those from manual homes show significant deficit. This trend is not due to differences in weight distribution between the three groups since there is little variation between mean birth weight scores. Mean birth weight for LBW in Classes I – IIIa is 2173 g compared with 2190 g for those in Classes IIIb and c and 2112 g for those in Classes IV and V. A beneficial environment therefore may modify intellectual deficit. On the other hand, part of the reason for the deficit in the manual classes could be due to the finding that these classes were least well matched in terms of sociological status and socio-cultural and economic background (see Chapter 4).

For both LBW and controls, the least number of Bender errors are scored by those children from Classes I – IIIa and most by those from Classes IV and V. Degree of impairment, however, is fairly constant between all three groups with those from Classes I – IIIa and IV and V showing the largest differences (Figure 7.8d). Once again, integration errors contributed most to this deficit and a marked impairment is apparent for these same groups (Figure 7.8e). While LBW of Social Classes IIIb and c showed a non-significant deficit of 0.23 points, those from I – IIIa and IV and V made significantly more errors of integration (0.46 and 0.47, respectively). This would suggest that LBW children from the extremes of the social spectrum have incurred neurological damage while those in the middle are relatively free of such handicap. Our neurological ratings (Table 7.18) support this view. Those LBW children from Classes I – IIIa, in particular, but also those from IV and V, include a greater number considered to have MBD or more severe abnormality than their controls (28 per cent LBW compared to 7 per cent controls in Classes I – IIIa and 28 per cent LBW and 18 per cent controls in Classes IV and V). Though the most significant disparity has occurred in Classes IIIb and c, this was due to more LBW having a doubtful rating. In terms of the number considered to show definite neurological impairment, little difference is noted (12 per cent LBW compared to 8 per cent controls). LBW children then, from favourable homes, have not overcome neurological deficit. The finding that LBW children from skilled manual homes are least neurologically impaired does not appear to be related to the number of neonatal problems since these LBW had the most. However,

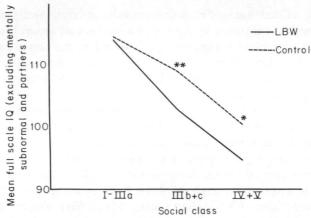

Figure 7.8a   Mean scores for Social Class groups: full IQ scale

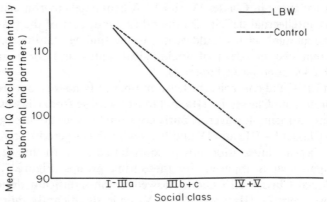

Figure 7.8b   Mean scores for Social Class groups: verbal IQ scale

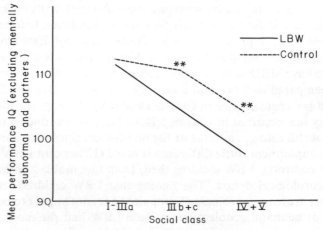

Figure 7.8c   Mean scores for Social Class groups: performance IQ scale

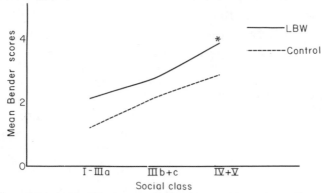

Figure 7.8d   Mean scores for Social Class groups: Bender scores

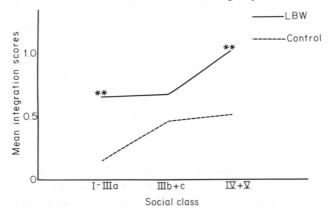

Figure 7.8e   Mean scores for Social Class groups: integration scores

although their mothers also had the poorest obstetric histories, few complications during pregnancy or delivery were noted. In contrast, mothers of LBW children from Classes I – IIIa tended to have more complications during pregnancy and delivery with mothers from the least skilled manual homes having had the worst general health during pregnancy.

To find out whether the noted relationship of birth weight and impairment, found for all LBW children, occurs in each social group, bivariate regressions of birth weight on impairment scores were performed within each social group. Figure 7.9a shows the three resulting regression lines for full IQ deficit. Birth weight has most effect on LBW from Classes IV and V, then I – IIIa, and, finally, has least effect on those from IIIb and c. The respective correlation coefficients of birth weight and IQ impairment are -0.328, -0.361, and -0.080 with only the former being significant (at 0.05 level). For the non-manual and unskilled

Table 7.18   Neurological ratings by social class. (Percentages in brackets)

Social Class	I – IIIa		IIIb and IIIc		IV – V	
	LBW	Control	LBW	Control	LBW	Control
Normal	14(50)	19(68)	23(50)	35(74)	27(48)	31(55)
Doubtful	6(21)	7(25)	18(38)	8(17)	13(25)	15(27)
MBD	4(14)	2(7)	5(10)	4(8)	8(14)	9(16)
More severe	4(14)	0(0)	1(2)	0(0)	8(14)	1(2)
Total	28(100)	28(100)	47(100)	47(100)	56(100)	56(100)
chi-square	0.139		0.057*		0.115	

Table 7.19   Mean impairment scores by social class and birth weight (excluding the mentally subnormal)

	Social Class I – IIIa		Social Class IIIb and IIIc		Social Class IV and V	
	$\leqslant$ 2000 g	> 2000 g	$\leqslant$ 2000 g	> 2000 g	$\leqslant$ 2000 g	> 2000 g
Full IQ scale	– 11.00**	+ 2.95	– 7.89	– 5.63*	– 13.75****	– 0.83
Bender score	+ 1.30	+ 0.67	+ 0.62	+ 0.48	+ 1.32	+ 0.91
Integration errors	+ 1.40**	+ 0.20	+ 0.50	+ 0.20	+ 0.40	+ 0.50*

manual classes, the correlations are stronger than those found for all LBW children, since a more homogeneous environment within the group has removed some of the variation in scores. For LBW children from the skilled manual classes, birth weight has had virtually no influence on subsequent impairment. Table 7.19, using mean impairment scores for each social group divided according to birth weight (above and below 2000 g), shows the same trends. The two groups of LBW children from the skilled manual classes show a similar degree of impairment, while for LBW from the extremes of the social spectrum the lighter LBW children show significant deficit and the heavier ones very little (LBW children from non-manual homes actually do better than their controls). Thus while, on average, a LBW child from Classes I – IIIa is unimpaired, those of very low birth weight show intellectual deficit in comparison with their controls. A favourable environment has not overcome the deleterious effects of very low birth weight, though they may have been modified since the deficit is less than for very low birth weight children from Classes IV and V. For the heavier LBW children, however, complete compensation has occurred since these children on average have higher IQ scores than their controls. While overall, similar intellectual deficit was noted for the two manual classes, it appears from our sample that, for the unskilled classes, birth weight is important in determining degree of deficit while for the skilled classes, actual weight in the LBW range is unimportant. For heavier LBW children, those from unskilled families are less impaired than those of skilled families while for lower weights (below 1500 g according to Figure 7.9a), the reverse is true. Part of the reason for these trends may be the difference in frequency of neonatal problems for each group. The disparity in IQ deficit parallels the disparity in the incidence of neonatal problems between birth weight groups in each social class. Lighter LBW infants in I – IIIa and IV – V had considerably more problems than the heavier LBW, while less disparity is noted between birth weight groups in Classes IIIb and c.

Figure 7.9b shows the comparable regression lines for birth weight on Bender impairment. The lines for LBW children from Classes I – IIIa and IV and V are similar, with decreasing impairment noted as birth weight increases (as was found in the whole LBW sample). For LBW children of Classes IIIb and c, however, minimal impairment is predicted for all. Correlation coefficients for the three groups are -0.26 (IV and V), -0.21 (I – IIIa) and -0.001 (IIIb and c), none of which is significant, and which is negligible in the case of those in Classes IIIb and c. Rather than all LBW children of Classes IIIb and c showing impairment, the very low correlation coefficient indicates that Bender impairment scores for this group of LBW children has been very random over the whole LBW range. Table 7.19 shows the mean Bender impairment scores for each social group. None of the differences are statistically significant but, again, least deficit on average is noted in Social Classes IIIb and c. Mean integration deficit scores are also shown in Table 7.19, revealing a similar degree of deficit between birth weight groups for the manual classes, while the lightest LBW group from the non-manual classes shows a highly significant degree of deficit. The infants in this group did not appear to have any more neonatal problems than those lighter LBW infants in other social groups. Their mothers, however, had the greatest frequency of complications during pregnancy and had poor obstetric histories. The significant deficit, then, found for all LBW in Classes I – IIIa and IV and V is attributable to the lightest weight group in the non-manual classes but is evenly distributed over both birth weight groups for those in the unskilled manual classes.

Our neurological ratings (Table 7.20) show significant neurological deficit for the lighter LBW groups in both the non-manual and skilled manual classes, while the heavier LBW groups in these classes have little disparity. (In I – IIIa, 62 per cent lighter LBW compared with 0 per cent controls and in IIIb and c, 22 per cent LBW and 0 per cent controls are rated as having MBD or more severe abnormality. Comparable figures in the heavier weight groups are 15 per cent and 10 per cent for those in I – IIIa and 10 per cent and 10 per cent for those in IIIb and c.) In the unskilled manual classes, a similar degree of deficit is noted

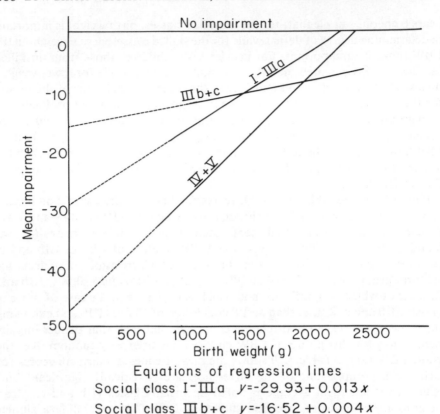

Equations of regression lines

Social class I-IIIa $y = -29.93 + 0.013x$

Social class IIIb+c $y = -16.52 + 0.004x$

Social class IV+V $y = -46.42 + 0.019x$

Figure 7.9a   Regression of birth weight on impairment scores for each social group: full IQ scale

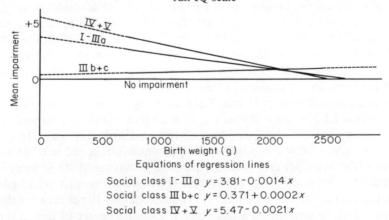

Equations of regression lines

Social class I-IIIa $y = 3.81 - 0.0014x$

Social class IIIb+c $y = 0.371 + 0.0002x$

Social class IV+V $y = 5.47 - 0.0021x$

Figure 7.9b   Regression of birth weight on impairment scores for each social group: Bender score

Table 7.20 Neurological ratings by social class and birth weight. (Percentages in brackets)

Social Class	I – IIIa				IIIb – IIIc				IV – V			
	≤2000	Control	>2000	Control	≤2000	Control	>2000	Control	≤2000	Control	>2000	Control
Normal	2(25)	6(75)	12(60)	13(65)	3(33)	8(89)	20(53)	27(71)	10(48)	11(52)	17(49)	20(57)
Doubtful	1(12)	2(25)	5(25)	5(25)	4(44)	1(11)	14(37)	7(18)	5(24)	6(29)	8(23)	9(20)
MBD	3(37)	0(0)	1(5)	2(10)	2(22)	0(0)	3(8)	4(10)	3(14)	4(19)	5(14)	5(14)
More severe	2(25)	0(0)	2(10)	0(0)	0(0)	0(0)	1(2)	0(0)	3(14)	0(0)	5(14)	1(3)
Total	8(100)	8(100)	20(100)	20(100)	9(100)	9(100)	38(100)	38(100)	21(100)	21(100)	35(100)	35(100)
chi-square	0.025**		0.499		0.048**		0.211		0.035		0.397	

in both weight groups (comparable figures are 28 per cent and 19 per cent in the lighter LBW group and 28 per cent and 17 per cent in the heavier group). While neurological impairment is equally prevalent for both weight groups in the unskilled manual classes, for the other LBW children, the lighter LBW children exhibit more impairment and this is particularly evident in those from the non-manual classes.

CONCLUSION

In accordance with the majority of previous studies using similar LBW samples, our LBW group had a greater incidence of mental and educational subnormality than their matched controls and exhibited impairment in intelligence, perceptuomotor skills, academic performance, and behaviour ratings. Our lighter LBW children (2000 g and below) tended to contribute most to the noted deficits. Amongst the heavier LBW children, only the 'growth-retarded prematures' exhibited intellectual impairment. Growth retardation, regardless of gestational age, appears to produce a deficit in the integrative function of perception and our evidence suggests that the male is especially susceptible. Children of the non-manual classes showed least intellectual impairment, though this may be partly due to better matching with their controls in terms of socio-economic status. The extremes of the social spectrum incurred most neurological deficit: for the unskilled manual classes this deficit was noted in both birth weight groups, while for the non-manual group it was found to be particularly prevalent in the lighter LBW children.

ABBREVIATIONS USED IN CHAPTER 7

GA	Gestational Age
FBW	Full Birth Weight, i.e. above LBW limit
LBW	Low Birth Weight
Prem.	Premature
AFD	Appropriate for Dates
SFD	Small for Dates
LFD	Light for Dates
Bayley	Bayley Scales of Mental and Motor Development
Bender	Bender Gestalt Test of Visual Motor Co-ordination
BSAG	Bristol Social Adjustment Guide
Gesell	Gesell Developmental Scale
Goodenough	Goodenough 'Draw a Person' Test
Griffith	Griffith Developmental Scale
ITPA	Illinois Test of Psycholinguistic Abilities
Lincoln Oseretsky	Lincoln Oseretsky Test of Motor Development

SB	Stanford Binet Intelligence Scale
Vineland	Vineland Social Maturity Scale
WISC	Wechsler Intelligence Scale for Children
WPPSI	Wechsler Preschool and Primary Scales of Intelligence
WRAT	Wide Range Achievement Test

Low Birth Weight: A Medical, Psychological, and Social Study
Edited by R. Illsley and R.G. Mitchell
© 1984 John Wiley & Sons Ltd

Chapter 8

The Follow-up Study: Medical Aspects

J. CATER AND M. GILL

All the children in the study sample who were available for examination at the 10 year follow-up—a total of 282 children (143 LBW and 139 controls)—were medically examined by one of us (MG). The examination, which included general physical and neurological components, was carried out on a date as near the child's tenth birthday as possible. The examiner had no knowledge of the children's histories before the examinations, which were undertaken mainly in school (262) but occasionally in hospital (4 inpatients and 7 outpatients), at home (6) or at the Institute of Medical Sociology (3). The children were usually unaccompanied but a parent or nurse was present when there was a specific problem such as mental or physical disability.

Each examination took at least 45 minutes and was conducted as informally as possible, the added advantage of being in familiar surroundings helping to ensure good co-operation from the children. If anything was discovered which required further action, the child was referred either to the family doctor or to the school health officer.

GENERAL PHYSICAL EXAMINATION

Methods and procedure

Body measurements

The growth of LBW children being of particular interest, the examination began with the measurement of height, weight, and head circumference. To avoid inconsistencies in measurement due to variations in the equipment used in the schools, the examiner carried her own scale, ruler, and measuring tape. Height was measured with the child standing on the floor with heels and back against the wall, the neck being stretched slightly by the examiner and a rule placed on the head. The children were weighed in their underpants on a Krups personal weighing scale which was carried by the examiner and checked regularly. Head circumference was measured by taking the maximal occipito-frontal circumference. All three measurements were charted on Tanner/Whitehouse 1959 centile charts.

Puberty rating

To ascertain whether there was any difference in the sexual development of LBW children, the development of the breasts and genitalia and the presence of pubic and axillary hair were rated on the Tanner scale, which ranges from pre-adolescent development at Stage 1 to full adult development at Stage 5 (Tanner, 1962).

Minor anomalies

During the examination, record was made of any minor physical abnormalities, such as low set ears, slanting palpebral fissures, abnormal palmar creases and so on.

As emphasized by Drillien and Drummond (1977), certain combinations of minor anomalies should alert the examiner to look for a specific disorder such as Down's Syndrome or, as was the case in this study, the Rubinstein-Taybi Syndrome.

Findings of general examination

Body measurements

LBW children were lighter and shorter and had smaller head circumferences than control children.

1. The mean body weight of the LBW children (28.3 kg) was significantly less ($p = 0.01$) than that of the control group (30.2 kg), a difference of 1.9 kg (Table 8.1). The difference was even greater (2.9 kg) for children weighing between 740 and 2000 g at birth (Table 8.2).
2. The mean height of LBW children was 3.3 cm less than that of their controls ($p = 0.001$) and again the difference between LBW and control groups was greater (6.1 cm) for children of birth weight 2000 g or less (Tables 8.1 and 8.2).

Table 8.1 Medical findings at 10-year follow-up of LBW and control children

	LBW	Controls	Significance (p value)
Body weight in kg (mean and S.D.)	28.3 ± 4.8	30.2 4.7	0.01
Height in cm (mean and S.D.)	132.1 8.1	135.4 5.1	0.001
Head circumference in cm (mean and S.D.)	53.1 1.6	53.8 1.6	0.001
Systolic blood pressure in mmHg (mean and S.D.)	112.7 9.4	107.3 9.9	0.001
Diastolic blood pressure in mmHg (mean and S.D.)	73.8 7.1	70.5 8.2	0.001
Visual acuity (% abnormal)	31.7	16.7	0.001
Strabismus (% abnormal)	12.5	3.9	0.03
Blow out cheeks (% abnormal)	5.2	0	0.002
Tendon reflexes (% abnormal)	33.3	20.1	0.04
Plantar response (% abnormal)	10.4	4.5	NS
Co-ordination (% abnormal)	6.7	0.7	0.03
Hands outstretched (% abnormal)	31.3	20.6	0.07
Soft neurological signs (% with score 2 or more)	67.4	64.4	NS

Table 8.2 Medical findings at 10-year follow-up of children of birth weight 740–2000 g and controls

	LBW	Controls	Significance (p value)
Body weight in kg (mean and S.D.)	27.2 4.6	30.1 4.3	0.02
Height in cm (mean and S.D.)	130.6 11.9	136.7 4.5	0.01
Head circumference in cm (mean and S.D.)	52.7 1.4	54.1 1.3	0.001
Systolic blood pressure in mmHg (mean and S.D.)	111.7 9.0	107.1 8.4	0.05
Diastolic blood pressure in mmHg (mean and S.D.)	74.3 7.1	70.6 7.5	0.05
Visual acuity (% abnormal)	40.5	10.8	0.005
Tendon reflexes (% abnormal)	48.7	20.5	0.03
Plantar response (% abnormal)	17.9	2.6	0.08
Hands outstretched (% abnormal)	38.9	16.7	0.03
Soft neurological signs (% with score 2 or more)	71.6	66.7	0.04

3. The mean occipito-frontal circumference of the LBW children (53.1 cm) was slightly smaller than that of the control group (53.8 cm). The difference is highly significant statistically but its clinical importance is dubious.

The measurements for body weight and height of the control children were very similar to those of the general population, the centile frequency distribution being identical to that of the Tanner/Whitehouse 1959 standards. In contrast, two-thirds of the whole sample, LBW and controls, had head circumferences above the 50th centile.

Puberty rating

Only 34 per cent of the LBW children had started puberty, compared with 49.6 per cent of the control children. The highest proportion of non-pubertal children was amongst those weighing 740 to 2000 gm at birth. When pubertal changes were present, they were more advanced in the control children: thus grade 3 changes were noted in 13.3 per cent of controls and only 3.7 per cent of LBW children. The relationship of puberty to growth is well known and in part accounts for the differences in growth between the LBW children and their controls. Many factors contribute to the onset of puberty and it is not possible to identify the particular effect of low weight at birth.

Minor anomalies

Minor physical abnormalities were noted more frequently amongst the LBW children and were of great variety. Those most noteworthy were unusual palpebral fissures (17 LBW, 4 control, $p = 0.012$), abnormalities in the shape of the neck (4 LBW, 0 control, $p = 0.029$), and umbilical or inguinal hernias (7 LBW, 3 control, $p = 0.21$).

Lymphadenopathy

Slight generalized enlargement of lymph nodes was more frequently observed amongst the LBW children than amongst their controls. While not of great clinical importance, this may reflect a higher incidence of infection in the LBW group.

Blood pressure

Both systolic and diastolic pressures were consistently higher in the LBW children than in their controls (Tables 8.1 to 8.3). Although the differences are statistically significant the variation is unlikely to be important clinically and may partly be due to the greater level of anxiety noted amongst the LBW children.

Table 8.3   Medical findings at 10-year follow-up of children of birth weight
2001–2500 g and controls

	LBW		Controls		Significance (p value)
Body weight in kg (mean and S.D.)	28.6	4.9	30.2	4.8	0.005
Height in cm (mean and S.D.)	132.6	5.8	134.6	5.4	0.02
Systolic blood pressure in mmHg (mean and S.D.)	113.0	9.5	107.4	10.4	0.0001
Diastolic blood pressure in mmHg (mean and S.D.)	73.6	7.0	70.5	8.5	0.01
Visual acuity (% abnormal)	27.7		19.3		0.04

NEUROLOGICAL EXAMINATION

Methods and procedure

A full neurological examination was carried out on each child. During this, the emotional state of the child was observed, e.g. any undue anxiety, and his behaviour was assessed, e.g. the degree of impulsiveness or overactivity displayed.

Speech

This was assessed only as normal or abnormal.

Cranial nerves

The following cranial nerves were tested.

II   The optic nerve. Visual acuity was tested using standard Snellen Charts or Stycar Letters and Toys (Sheridan 1976a). Colour vision was tested using Ishihara Plates, and the visual fields were determined by the confrontation method. Funduscopy was carried out with a surprising amount of co-operation considering the absence of any mydriatic.

III, IV, VI   The oculomotor, trochlear, and abducens nerves. Eye movements and pupillary reactions were tested and the presence of nystagmus, strabismus, or cataract noted.

V   The trigeminal nerve. The motor function of the fifth nerve was tested by asking the child to clench the jaw and the sensory function by means of cotton wool and pinprick (omitting the corneal reflex).

VII   The facial nerve. The child was asked to blow out his cheeks and any weakness was observed.

VIII The auditory nerve. Hearing was tested by whispering numbers at distances up to twenty feet, or with cup, paper, and rattle in the case of the handicapped child (Sheridan 1976b). Audiometric reports were subsequently obtained from school records for 270 of the children.

XII The hypoglossal nerve. The tongue was observed for wasting or fasciculation and any deviation from the mid-line when protruded.

Motor and reflex functions

Posture and gait were observed and any involuntary movements noted. The mass, power and tone of the muscles were determined and tendon reflexes elicited. Evidence of lack of co-ordination was sought by using tests such as the finger-to-nose test, the fingers-thumb test and maintenance of posture tests (Paine and Oppé, 1966; Touwen and Prechtl, 1970).

Sensory function

Touch, position sense, and vibration were tested by standard methods. Specific tests of cortical sensory function were carried out, viz.: recognition of objects, graphaesthesia, and discrimination of two points (Paine and Oppé, 1966). Hand and foot dominance were recorded, as was the ability to discriminate between left and right (see below).

'Soft' signs

Low weight at birth is generally considered to be a factor in the aetiology of minimal brain dysfunction (MBD), about which many differing views have been expressed (Bax and Mac Keith, 1963; Touwen and Sporrel, 1979). There is a general agreement, however, that minor or 'soft' neurological signs can be elicited in certain children by using specific tests of visual perception and motor ability (Paine and Oppé, 1966; Schain, 1973). It was decided therefore to use some of these 'soft' signs, in conjunction with a clinical appraisal of the child's behaviour during the medical examination, as a basis for comparison with the psychological tests and the school teacher's report. The tests chosen were as follows:

1. Object recognition. Five objects—a bottle top, a coin, a button of similar size, a key, and a block—were placed in the hand one at a time. The time taken for recognition and any error in identification were recorded.
2. Graphaesthesia. The numbers 1, 8, and 0 had to be recognised when written on the palm of the hand with a pencil.
3. Two point discrimination. The points of a paper clip were placed on the skin 2 mm apart on the fingers and lips, 10—20 mm apart on the face and 20—30 mm apart on the dorsum of the foot.

A normal response to these three tests of cortical sensory function requires integration of the sensations of touch and pressure and the ability to recognise. Like Touwen and Prechtl (1970), the examiner found difficulty in the interpretation of the results of the test for two point discrimination.

4. Finger-to-nose test. The tip of the index finger was placed on the tip of the nose when the eyes were open and then when the eyes were closed.
5. Fingers-to-thumb test. The fingers of one hand were placed consecutively on the thumb of the same hand as quickly as possible.
6. Pronation/supination. The hand and forearm were rapidly pronated and supinated.
7. Maintenance of posture. The child stood with feet together and arms outstretched and was then asked to close his eyes.
8. Heel-toe walking. The child walked along a straight line placing one foot directly in front of the other.
9. Test 8 was repeated with eyes closed.
10. Hopping. The child was asked to hop on each foot 20 times.
11. Laterality. Hand preference was tested by asking the child to write his name, and foot preference by asking him to kick a football or hop.
12. Right and left discrimination. This was tested by asking the child to touch his left ear and stick up his right thumb. He was then asked to point to the examiner's left ear and right thumb. Mixed laterality and failure to discriminate between left and right are more common in children with any kind of organic brain syndrome (Paine and Oppé, 1966, Schain, 1973).

The findings were scored and the results, together with the assessment of mental state and behaviour, were compared with the psychological tests and the teacher's report. After discussion with the psychologist, a judgement was reached as to whether or not the diagnosis of MBD could be made, while at the same time recognizing the limitations of this term (Touwen and Sporrel, 1979).

Findings of neurological examination

The main purpose of the neurological examination was to identify two groups of children: those in whom a firm diagnosis of a neurological disorder could be made and those with signs consistent with the diagnosis of MBD. Differences in the incidence of certain neurological signs indicating possible abnormality were also recorded.

Neurological sequelae

In the years following birth, cerebral palsy was diagnosed in 6 of the LBW children: mild spastic diplegia in 2, minimal spastic monoplegia in 1, and mixed forms of cerebral palsy in 3. Other abnormalities found were Rubinstein-Taybi syndrome (1 child), epiloia (1 child), and blindness with deafness due to intra-

Table 8.4   Abnormal physical and neurological findings in the sample

Case no.	Birth weight	Cerebral palsy	Other conditions	IQ
LBW group				
5	740	Mixed	Retrolental fibroplasia, epilepsy, and scoliosis	Not scored
21	2100	No	Epiloia	Not scored
24	1900	Diplegia	Epilepsy	Not scored
26	2040	Monoplegia	Poor vision	70
35	2180	No	Increased soft CNS signs	64
52	2030	No	Blind and deaf	85
91	2100	Diplegia		110
92	2180	No	Increased soft CNS signs	60
93	1660	Mixed		62
100	1016	No	Increased soft CNS signs	114
102	1930	No	Increased soft CNS signs	69
113	2400	No	Rubinstein−Taybi syndrome	61
131	2175	Mixed		Not scored
Control group				
527	3020	No	Increased soft CNS signs	

uterine rubella (1 child). Thus the expected excess of neurological disorders amongst LBW children was confirmed (Table 8.4). The comparatively low rates of cerebral palsy and mental handicap are consistent with the findings of other studies of LBW children undertaken at the same period.

Visual acuity

Vision was considered to be normal in 45 per cent of the LBW group and 69 per cent of the controls. Impaired visual acuity (vision of 12/60 or less in at least one eye) was found more frequently in LBW children (31.7 per cent) than in controls (16.7 per cent) and was especially common (40.5 per cent) amongst LBW children weighing 2000 g or less at birth (Tables 8.1 and 8.2).

Audiometry

Audiometric reports were obtained for 270 of the children in the sample. Grade I hearing deficit (loss of up to 35 decibels) was reported in 5 LBW children and 6 of the control group: the hearing loss was bilateral in 1 and 3 of these groups respectively. Grade II hearing loss (35−70 decibels) was found in 4 LBW and 2 control children. Hearing aids were worn by two of the LBW children and one of the controls. Definitive high tone deafness and conductive loss was identified in two LBW and 3 control children.

'Soft' neurological signs

A composite score was created by adding together the scores for the 12 neurological items listed above. Rather surprisingly, such soft signs were quite frequently recorded in the control population, 64 per cent showing two or more signs at the age of 10 years (Table 8.1). Slightly more of the LBW children showed these soft signs, the difference from the controls being statistically significant only in the 740–2000 g weight category (Tables 8.1 and 8.2: the totals, of course, include the children with cerebral palsy). The significance of this finding is difficult to assess. A substantial excess of soft signs (more than 5) was recorded in 4 LBW children and 1 control but in each case this was an isolated phenomenon and the children concerned were all functioning satisfactorily otherwise (Table 8.4).

Other neurological signs

1. *Tendon reflexes* Variations from normal were recorded almost twice as frequently amongst the LBW children (33.3 per cent LBW, 20.1 per cent controls) and most commonly amongst children who weighed 2000 g or less at birth (Tables 8.1 and 8.2).
2. *Plantar response* An extensor response is generally held to indicate neurological abnormality. However, it was elicited in 4.5 per cent of controls and 10.4 per cent of LBW children. The rate was substantially higher in LBW children who weighed 2000 g or less at birth (Table 8.2).
3. *Co-ordination* Abnormalities of co-ordination were noted in a small proportion of the LBW children (6.7 per cent LBW, 0.7 per cent controls). They did not bear any relationship to the category of low birth weight.
4. *Hands outstretched* The test with hands outstretched was unsatisfactorily performed by more of the LBW children (31.3 per cent LBW, 20.6 per cent controls, $p = 0.07$).

Comment

The expected excess of neurological disorders amongst LBW children was confirmed. Twice as many LBW as control children were assessed as having some kind of neurological abnormality (23 per cent LBW, 12 per cent controls). The excess in the LBW group comprised mainly the more severe forms of disorder, e.g. cerebral palsy or mental handicap, which were recorded in 9.9 per cent of the LBW group and 0.8 per cent of the controls.

Outcome for babies weighing less than 1501 g at birth

The survival rate for babies weighing less than 1501 g at birth has greatly improved following advances in neonatal intensive care. Their neurodevelopmental status is of particular interest because of the lingering fear that damaged children who would formerly have died may now survive to become the handicapped of the future.

Of the 13 such babies in our study, 4 were excluded from the follow-up analysis of matched pairs (see Chapter 6). One of these 4 could not be traced at 10 years, whereas the other 3 were medically examined and underwent intelligence tests but their controls could not be traced. Of these 3, 2 were physically normal and of average intelligence while the third, though well grown, had an IQ of only 72.

Thus 9 of these very small infants were included in the follow-up. At 10 years, 1 was a very small child (height 65 cm, weight 17 kg) who had mental retardation, epilepsy, retrolental fibroplasia, and mixed cerebral palsy. A second child had 7 minor neurological signs but was functioning normally physically and mentally. The neurodevelopmental status of the remainder was satisfactory.

In this group of 9 children, neonatal problems, apart from colour changes in 5, had been few. Assisted ventilation for respiratory distress syndrome had been given to 1, bicarbonate therapy to another, and a third had had severe progressive hypoglycaemia (this was the child with mental retardation, epilepsy and cerebral palsy mentioned above).

Outcome for children excluded from the follow-up study

Details of the 14 pairs of children excluded (see Chapter 6) are shown in Table 8.5. Of this group, 8 LBW and 4 control children were examined. All but one were considered to be normal apart from minor variations: the one abnormal child who was in the LBW group had an IQ less than 75. Minor variations recorded in the LBW group were a slightly large head in one child and hyperreflexia in another. Of the 4 controls, 1 showed hyperreflexia and 1 had a number of soft neurological signs.

The only child in the whole study who died was one of the LBW group.

Table 8.5 Outcome of children excluded from study (14 pairs)

	LBW	Controls
Normal	7	4
IQ less than 75	1	—
Not examined	6*	10

* 1 LBW child died.

INCIDENCE OF DISEASE RECORDED AT THE TEN YEAR FOLLOW-UP

The medical records of the Royal Aberdeen Children's Hospital were scrutinized for attendances of the 107 LBW children and their controls who, as far as was known, had lived in the RACH catchment area throughout their lives. The medical information so obtained is described under the eight headings that follow.

Respiratory disease

Referral to hospital for a specific respiratory disorder was not frequent (7 LBW, 3 control). Diagnoses included asthma, bronchitis, pneumonia, and croup.

Tonsillectomy

Operation to remove the tonsils and adenoids had been carried out on 18 LBW children and 10 controls: this difference probably reflects poorer health and increased parental anxiety in the LBW group.

Heart murmurs

A significant cardiac murmur was diagnosed by 10 years of age in 1 LBW and 1 control child. An 'innocent' murmur had been recognised before the age of 5 years in 10 LBW and 5 control children. A previous report from this study (Cater, 1978) noted that 2 LBW children and none of the controls were considered to have an organic murmur before the age of 4 years. These apparent discrepancies are in fact compatible, since it is well known that murmurs change in the early years of life and some defects, such as ventricular septal defects, close spontaneously.

Orthopaedic disorders

Congenital dislocation of the hip is an important condition in the newborn infant which tends to be over-diagnosed. Of the sample, 33 LBW infants and 13 controls had been recorded as having 'clicking hips' in the newborn period. Short term splinting was required by 11 LBW and 6 control infants but only 2 LBW children needed long term treatment. The only other notable condition found was Perthes disease in 2 control children.

Convulsions

A history of convulsions was more common amongst the LBW children at the 10 year survey (8 LBW, 1 control).

Visual disorders

Myopia, hypermetropia, strabismus, and astigmatism were mentioned in the hospital records of the LBW group much more frequently than in those of the control children (18 LBW, 6 control). This confirms other reports of an increased incidence of visual problems amongst LBW children.

Other disorders

A history of hernia (umbilical and inguinal) was noted in 10 LBW children and 3 controls. Enuresis was reported in 11 LBW and 7 control children, encopresis only in 2 of the LBW group. Miscellaneous referrals for symptoms such as headache occurred more frequently amongst the LBW group (12 LBW, 4 control).

Admission to hospital

LBW children were more often admitted to hospital than the controls (LBW 94 admissions, controls 58). The admission rate for surgical procedures was approximately the same in the two groups, so that the excess of admissions in the LBW group was mainly for medical disorders.

ATTENDANCE AT ACCIDENT AND EMERGENCY UNIT

Attendance at the Accident and Emergency Unit (AEU) of the Royal Aberdeen Children's Hospital was considered for the 86 pairs of children who, as far as was known, had always lived in the Aberdeen District, i.e. within easy travelling distance of the hospital. This restriction was made because children living further afield would generally have been seen by their family doctor in the first instance.

Over the 10-year period, use of the AEU was similar in the two groups: thus 67 LBW children accounted for 201 attendances and 66 control children attended a total of 190 times. In the first 5 years, 39 LBW children attended 69 times, compared with 46 control children who paid 104 visits to the AEU, the excess in the control group being mainly due to head injuries and burns. After the age of 5 years the situation was reversed, since 58 LBW and 48 control children accounted for 132 and 87 attendances respectively.

Analysis by social class showed that about 40 per cent of both LBW and control children from all social classes attended the AEU on one or two occasions in the 10-year period. Within each social class numbers of attendances were similar but there were striking differences between social classes. Thus in Social Classes I, II, and IIIa there were 15 pairs of children: 8 LBW and 9 control children had attended the AEU at some time; whereas 7 and 6, respectively, had never attended. By contrast, of 42 pairs in Social Classes IV and V, 35 LBW children had attended (10 of them five times or more), while 37 control children had attended (9 of them five times or more). Thus of the LBW sample, 53 per cent in Social Classes I–IIIa had attended the AEU compared with 83 per cent in Social Classes IV–V: the comparable figures for the controls were 60 and 88 per cent respectively.

SIGNIFICANCE OF PERINATAL EVENTS FOR
LATER HEALTH STATUS

In earlier sections of this chapter, the relationship of birth weight to growth and development and to medical disorders was examined. Here we consider the relationship of perinatal events to subsequent progress. Many aspects of this relationship were examined but the comparatively low incidence of physical abnormality at 10 years of age meant that, for most items, no significant association could be demonstrated. Moreover, the birth weight/gestational age sub-groups defined in Chapter 5 (page 95) did not prove useful for this analysis because of the relatively small numbers of children in some of the sub-groups. For the present purpose, therefore, we have considered the LBW sample mainly in the three birth weight categories used as the basis for the earlier analyses in this chapter, viz. the whole sample, those with birth weight between 740 and 2000 g and those with birth weight 2001 to 2500 g, although reference to the sub-groups is made where appropriate.

Nutrition

Intra-uterine growth retardation

The effects of fetal growth patterns on stature at 10 years were not particularly striking. The mean height of growth retarded infants was 3.6 cm less than that of their controls at 10 years, but comparable disparity occurred in the very premature and premature sub-groups (3.1 cm). However, the mean weight of the growth retarded premature LBW children was substantially less (by 3.2 kg) than that of their controls.

Postnatal nutrition

Poor nutrition as reflected in delayed regaining of birth weight and subsequent poor weight gain in early infancy may have important consequences for subsequent mental and physical development. Thus Drillien (1964) suggested that delayed start of feeding was important in the genesis of later disability in her LBW children who took longer to regain their birth weight. In the present study, sufficient detailed information about feeding in the early weeks was available for 77 LBW children. The mean IQ for this group was very much the same as for their controls.

Apgar scores

A weak positive association between extensor plantar responses and low Apgar scores at both 1 and 5 minutes was noted but numbers were too small for statistical analysis.

Biochemical changes

High bilirubin levels seldom occurred in the study sample and when they did they were controlled by exchange transfusion. Mean IQ ratings were the same irrespective of the neonatal bilirubin level in the plasma.

Hypoglycaemia, defined as a level of blood glucose below 20 mg% (1.1 mmol/1), was associated with low intelligence. Two profoundly mentally retarded children (both LBW) were considered to be handicapped as a result of neonatal hypoglycaemia.

Increase in the packed red cell volume (PCV) of capillary blood was not associated with later medical disorder amongst the children in our sample.

SIGNIFICANCE OF SEX AND SOCIAL CLASS

Sex of the child

Analysis at 10 years by sex of the child failed to show any significant differences apart from stature. The LBW group as a whole were shorter and lighter than their controls: LBW girls were similar in weight to their controls but shorter in stature.

Social class

The importance of social class for a variety of features in the follow-up study was examined, but only pubertal development showed an association of any significance. At the age of 10 years, none of the LBW or control children from manual occupational backgrounds (Social Classes IIIb, IV and V) had reached puberty. In the non-manual occupational groups (Social Classes I, II, and IIIa), more control than LBW children had reached puberty and more were at an advanced stage ($p = 0.02$).

An excess of children with enlarged lymph nodes was noted amongst both LBW and control children from social classes IV and V, presumably reflecting a greater incidence of infection in this disadvantaged group.

CONCLUSIONS FROM THE TEN YEAR MEDICAL FOLLOW-UP

1. The LBW children were shorter and lighter than the control children. Onset of puberty was later and pubertal changes advanced less quickly in the LBW group.
2. Abnormal neurological findings were more common in the LBW group.
3. In all these respects, children who weighed 2000 g or less at birth were at a disadvantage compared with heavier LBW children.

4. A very high proportion of audiometric reports was obtained for the children: the incidence of hearing loss was remarkably low.
5. A study of hospital records indicated that there was an excess of disease amongst the LBW group.
6. Simple comparison of the LBW and control groups showed no important association between perinatal events and health status at 10 years of age, apart from an association between neonatal hypoglycaemia and later mental handicap.

Low Birth Weight: A Medical, Psychological, and Social Study
Edited by R. Illsley and R.G. Mitchell
© 1984 John Wiley & Sons Ltd

Chapter 9

The Influence of Factors Associated with Low Birth Weight on Development at the Age of 10 Years

R. CARR-HILL, C. FRASER AND M. RUSSELL

INTRODUCTION

The sociological and medical factors associated with low weight at birth have been presented and discussed in Chapters 4 and 5, respectively. Chapters 7 and 8 described the developmental tests and medical examination which were carried out on the children at the age of 10 years and showed that there were considerable differences between the LBW children and their controls. The purpose of this chapter is to study the link, if any, between the two sets of findings; that is, to study the conjoint and relative power of medical (physiological) and sociological factors associated with being born at a low weight in predicting outcomes at age 10. Specifically, we shall be examining two broad questions:

1. Are any of the biological and social criteria studied at birth closely associated with the mental and physical development of the LBW children?
2. If so, do initial differences between the LBW and control groups explain any of the observed impairment among the LBW children?

These questions are designed to construct a predictive model, which could be of use in indicating, at the time of birth, which infants may be at risk of later impairment: this model can only partly account for any observed impairment, since our intermediate data on environmental influences during the first 10 years of life are insufficient to determine the extent to which they may have affected the growth and mental development of the children.

The following section discusses the methodology and techniques used to explore these two questions, while the substantive results concerning the factors influencing the mental and physical development of the LBW children are considered on page 218 and the analysis of the factors influencing impairment on page 235.

METHODOLOGY AND TECHNIQUES

The Model

The hypotheses which motivated the study relate to the mental and physical development of LBW children as compared to other children. Schematically, this can be represented as shown in Figure 9.1.

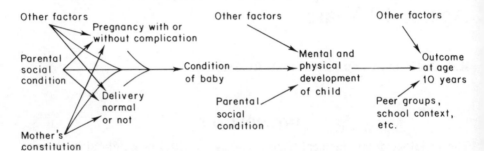

Figure 9.1   Factors affecting the mental and physical development of children

The first step in testing the model is to specify precisely the outcome variables. In this study we have selected eight attributes at age 10.

1. Full IQ
2. Verbal IQ
3. Performance IQ
4. Bender
5. Bender integration errors
6. Height in cm
7. Weight in kg
8. Head circumference in cm

These eight outcome variables fall into three groups, those related to mental development or IQ (1 to 3), those related to psychomotor development (4 and 5), and those related to physical development (6 to 8).

The next step is to specify the nature of the independent variables. In this study medical information has been collected on the pregnancy, the delivery, and the baby, and an interview was held with the mother to collect socio-cultural information about the family. As discussed elsewhere, we made no systematic collection of data on environmental influences during the first 10 years. In any case it would have been difficult to decide what information to collect. The breadth and range of data which would be required to fill out the parts of the 'model' referring to, for example, 'Peer Groups, School Context' is potentially vast.*

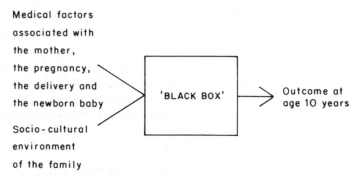

Figure 9.2   Schematic model indicating lack of information about environmental influences during childhood

It is not, therefore, appropriate to use the model in Figure 9.1 as our reference and that shown in Figure 9.2 is preferable, the 'black box' indicating an area devoid of information. This diagram represents the kind of model that can be tested with our data. There is one further complication in that, because we have conducted a matched case-control study, we are not testing a model over the whole possible range of babies, but a model for LBW babies as compared to control babies, the latter selected according to five matching variables. Indeed, one of the reasons for this design was the view that *separate models* might be appropriate for LBW and normal weight children: if this were the case then, although the simplistic schematization of Figure 9.2 would apply for both, the values of the parameters would be different for the two populations. In this mode, the dependent variables are the *values* of the eight outcome variables detailed above.

However, the same design also permits us to consider whether LBW is a *relative* handicap. Thus, we are searching for the *relative* effect of LBW as compared to the effects of other factors on later developmental outcome. In this latter model each pair of observations—on the case and its control—is treated as

* Thus in the controversy over the Coleman report (1966), the unanswerable criticisms were based on data that *ought* to have been gathered.

one so that the dependent variables are the *degree of impairment* of the LBW case relative to its control in respect of each of the outcome variables detailed above.

The variables

In building the model, four groups of variables are considered. Obviously, it is essential to include those sociological variables where the LBW and control groups differed: however, it is also important to consider the aetiological criteria for which the samples were matched, since some of these, e.g. social class and sex, are known to affect intelligence and growth, and so imperfections in matching might contribute to later differences in outcome between the two groups. The medical variables are also of two kinds: those which relate to the mother and are of aetiological importance in LBW, and which may have a direct or indirect physiological effect on the development of the child; and those which describe the physical condition of the baby at birth and reflect the degree of insult suffered before and during delivery, and which may affect subsequent development. The four groups of variables are therefore as follows:

Group 1 'Matching' variables—of known aetiological significance to LBW and child development.

Group 2 'Significant' sociological variables—where the LBW and control groups differ socially and therefore may be regarded as 'unmatched'.

Group 3 Maternal obstetric variables describing the health and physical status of the mother during pregnancy and delivery, and providing an index of previous reproductive performance.

Group 4 Neonatal variables describing the size, weight, gestational age and health status of the infant at birth.

The five matching variables in group 1 have been discussed in detail in Chapter 3. The choice of 'significant' sociological variables proved more difficult. The hospital interview survey elicited information over a very wide area, ranging from the socio-demographic characteristics of the parents to intended potty training habits. At the same time, the questions were rather too specific to the situation at birth. In Chapter 4, therefore, we have constructed indices which, we believe, better reflect the likely influence of sociological factors which differentiate between LBW and control children. The two sets of medical (physiological) variables were discussed in Chapter 5. The full set of variables is listed in Table 9.1: although these groups are eventually combined, so that the initial separation is not critical, it is useful from a theoretical perspective.

Techniques

Given the large number of variables involved, one of the families of

Table 9.1   Variables to be included in multiple regression analysis

Group 1 Matching criteria	Group 2 'Significant' sociological variables	Group 3 Maternal obstetric factors	Group 4 Neonatal variables
Social class Sex Maternal height Maternal smoking Parity	Mother's age (Indices of) Parental socio-cultural environment Parental recreational activities Parental expectations to influence Parental attitudes towards behaviour training Expected role of the husband Role preparation by the mother Interviewer's assessment of the mother	Pregnancy number Maternal delivery complications index Medical conditions specific to pregnancy index Medical complications of pregnancy index Previous obstetric history index	Birth weight Gestational age General nutritional status Neonatal problems index Number of days in special care unit (SCBU)

multivariate techniques is required. We have chosen multiple regression analysis to present the basic results. This method can typically be used in two ways. The first is as a predictive tool showing the extent to which variation in a dependent or outcome variable can be *accounted for* by variation in one or more independent or prior variables. In this approach the analysis demonstrates only whether or not variation in an independent variable or a set of independent variables makes a statistically significant contribution to variation in the outcome variable. The second approach, which is more informative, is to use the technique of multiple regression to provide estimates of the coefficients of a theoretically based model which links together *all* the relevant independent variables and the outcome(s) variable(s). In this approach the analysis concentrates on the *value* of (significant) coefficients, that is, the effect of a unit of change in an independent variable on the outcome variable.

However, this latter approach can only be used when the model has been specified in the design of the study. In this particular study, some important variables were not included, e.g. social circumstances during the 10-year period which makes it difficult to apply fully the second mode of analysis. For this reason we have tended to use multiple regression analysis as a predictive tool, so that more attention is paid to the significance of the coefficients rather than to their values. One exception should be noted: when differences in height are considered the value of the coefficient is crucial because of the peculiar nature of the differences in height variable (because height itself was used as a matching variable).

Multiple regression analysis provides an estimate of the contribution of each independent variable in predicting outcome scores, while simultaneously controlling for the influence of the other variables included in the analysis. This estimate is therefore a measure of the *independent* effect additional to the effects of the other variables included in the analysis. In other words it is important to note that, since the mechanics of any multivariate technique depend on the *deviations* or *squared deviations* from mean values, some constraints are imposed on the types of variables which can be included if we want to be able to interpret the estimates derived. Specifically the variables must all be treated as interval or binary in order that the differences between values can be interpreted: for example, 'social class'—a categorical or, for some writers, a ranked variable—was condensed into the two categories of manual and non-manual so that it could be analysed as a binary variable.

If we want to be confident in the standard errors of the estimates and, *a fortiori*, in the tests of significance for the coefficients, we have to be reasonably certain that the distribution of errors is not highly skewed. This is especially a problem with binary dependent variables. It would have been interesting, for example, to have used our neurological rating at 10 years as a dependent variable but this is a categorical variable and it would have to be transformed to an interval scale of 'degree of neurological impairment' which would present a whole range of problems. The alternative would be to assess children at age 10 as neurologically impaired or not which, besides being a dangerously prescriptive exercise, would have produced a very skew dependent variable.

Various statistics may be calculated in multiple regression, giving different types of information. The total contribution of the independent variables is expressed as 'R squared' (R^2) and is the amount of variance in the dependent variable which can be accounted for by the conjoint influence of all the independent variables in the analysis. The amount of independent influence each variable has is signified by the 'partial B' value and indicates how much one unit change in the independent variable will affect the dependent variable. Thus, for example, if independent variable A has a partial B value of 0.2 on dependent variable B, then 0.2 of a unit change in A will result in one unit change in B. Since the independent variables are measured by different units, partial B does not permit direct comparison of the relative effect of the different independent variables. For this reason the 'standardized partial B' was designed: its value indicates how much a change of one standard deviation in the independent variable will affect the dependent variable, controlling as before for all other variables in the regression analysis.

The foregoing gives only a summary account of multiple regression and readers who wish further details are advised to consult any standard statistical text (e.g. *Statistical Analysis of Social Data* by Zeller and Carmines, 1978).

At the same time, we have supplemented the findings from multiple regression with a discriminant analysis. This technique takes two (or more) exclusive groups defined *a priori* in terms of one or more criteria and searches for the variables which most distinguish between the groups. The major analytic difficulty is in deciding which of several possible distance measures should be used to determine the most effective discriminatory variables. Indeed it is partly because there is no conventional agreement on the appropriate distance measure that discriminant analysis is less widely used than multiple regression analysis but, in some situations, discriminant analysis provides a clearer picture of which factors are important. We have chosen to use a stepwise method of selecting independent variables for entry into the analysis based on Rao's V, a generalized distance measure. Thus, as we want to know what distinguishes between those who are impaired and those who are not, we have conducted the analysis in terms of two groups so defined for the three sets of scores (IQ, Bender, and physical).

Various statistics are produced in the course of computing the discriminant function, that is, the linear combination of variables which most effectively assigns observations to one or other of the two groups. We can compare the means and standard deviations of the independent variables for each group and the total set of cases; we can also compare the pooled within groups correlation and covariance matrices with the overall correlation and covariance matrices. Together these two comparisons help us to assess the effect of splitting the population this way on the form of the relationships between the variables. At each stage in the selection procedure, the algorithm calculates the partial multivariate F ratios for each variable not yet included in the discriminant function and at the same time conducts a one-way analysis of variance for the equality of group means on each of the discriminating variables. We shall be referring in the first instance to the order in which the variables enter the discriminant function and, secondly, to the values of the F ratios.

To recapitulate, the dependent variables are the mental scores (full, verbal, and performance IQ), the psycho-motor scores (Bender), and the physical measurements (height, weight, and head circumference) assessed when the children in the study were 10 years old. Our independent variables consist of the four groups of variables obtained around the time of birth. Thus, by conducting a multiple regression analysis of the dependent variable in terms of the independent variables, we should be able to ascertain which of the influences measured at birth have most effect in determining subsequent physical and mental development. And by conducting a discriminant analysis between groups defined in terms of these dependent variables, we can show which of the groups of variables most clearly distinguished between, for example, those children who are relatively most impaired and those who are not impaired.

Hypothesis

The earlier chapters have documented the medical and social differences and similarities between the LBW children and their controls both at birth and at the 10-year follow-up. The purpose of this chapter, as outlined above, is to put these differences and similarities into relation with one another and, specifically, to assess the relative contribution of medical and social differences at birth to the observed impairments at age 10. In order to follow the ensuing analysis it will be useful to repeat these main findings, drawing attention to those results which appear to be in conflict or just simply curious.

The study at birth showed that the LBW mothers were reproductively more inefficient, in the sense that they had more spontaneous abortions or induced terminations. These mothers had experienced more medical conditions specific to pregnancy such as pre-eclamptic toxaemia and haemorrhage and more medical complications such as anaemia, gynaecological disorders, and respiratory or other infections. During delivery, the LBW mothers had also experienced more premature rupture of the membranes, more obstetric intervention, and a longer labour (note that the proportions induced were the same). Finally, low Apgar scores were more frequent in the LBW than in the control group and the LBW children had lower blood pressure than the controls. On this basis five indices were constructed in Chapter 6: the previous obstetric history index, medical conditions specific to pregnancy index, general medical complications of pregnancy index, maternal complications of delivery index, and neonatal problems index, each of which discriminates between the LBW and control groups.

Moreover, among the LBW children, we can usefully distinguish between five birth weight centile/gestational age groups: the very premature (gestation < 32 weeks); growth-retarded prematures (LBW infant on or below 10th centile and with gestation between 32 and 36 weeks inclusive); premature (LBW infant above 10th centile and with gestation between 32 and 36 weeks inclusive); growth-retarded (all LBW infants on or below 10th centile with gestation 37 weeks or more); and small normals (all LBW infants above 10th centile with gestation 37 weeks or more). The following illustrate the utility of this distinction:

1. LBW infants who were lighter or born earlier had more neonatal problems than those who were heavier or born later irrespective of maternal histories and experiences;
2. While the very premature infants were less at risk from maternal illness, the premature infants tended to be born to mothers with the worst obstetric histories and LBW infants born at term were most at risk of complications of delivery.

The postnatal interview questionnaires yielded considerably more data but of a diffuse kind. For this reason, the analysis in Chapter 4 concentrated directly on the derivation of indices to reflect different domains of interest. Hence, we analysed the responses to the questionnaire in five groups and showed the following:

1. The socio-cultural background of the LBW families was on the whole poorer than the controls; moreover, their life-style in terms of entertainment and recreation was less varied.
2. The LBW mother had less aspirations and expectations for the development of her child than the control mother.
3. The LBW mother's attitude to behaviour training was more rigid than that of the control mother.
4. The LBW mother apportioned a slighter role to the husband in matters of child-rearing.
5. The LBW mother was less prepared for motherhood than the control mother.

Moreover, the interviewers' assessments of the mothers' range of vocabulary, fluency of expression, and organization clearly favoured the control mother.

The 10 year medical follow-up discussed in Chapter 8 showed the following:

1. The LBW children were shorter and lighter and had smaller heads than the control children. Onset of puberty was later and pubertal changes advanced less quickly in the LBW group.
2. Abnormal neurological findings were more common in the LBW group.
3. A very high proportion of audiometric reports was obtained for the LBW children: the incidence of hearing loss was remarkably low;
4. A study of hospital records indicated that there was an excess of disease amongst the LBW group.

We note also that in respect of most aspects of physical development, children who had weighed 2000 g or less at birth were at a disadvantage compared with heavier LBW children; and that the only important associations between perinatal events and health status was that between neonatal hypoglycaemia and later mental handicap.

The 10 year psychological examination discussed in Chapter 7 showed that:

1. The LBW group had a greater incidence of mental and educational sub-normality than their matched controls.
2. The LBW group were impaired in intelligence, perceptuo-motor skills, academic performance, and behaviour ratings.

We note also that the lighter LBW children (2000 g and below) tended to contribute most to the noted deficits and that, amongst the heavier LBW children, only the growth-retarded prematures exhibited intellectual impairment. Moreover, our non-manual children showed least intellectual impairment, though this may be partly due to better matching with their controls in terms of socio-economic status. The extremes of the social spectrum incurred most neurological deficit: for the unskilled manual classes this deficit was noted in both birth weight groups, while for the non-manual group it was found to be particularly prevalent in the lighter LBW children.

Weaving all this into a coherent set of hypotheses about the relationship between the differences and similarities at birth and the differences and similarities at age 10, which can then be tested within the framework of a model, is an impossible task for the reasons explained on page 208. However, we can suggest various lines of analysis that should be followed. First, it is clear that, both at birth and at age 10, not only are there important differences between growth retarded and premature LBW children at birth but the relationships between other factors at birth and outcomes at age 10 are also likely to be different. In particular, the role of neonatal problems is differentiated as between growth-retarded and premature children. Second, there are clear differences between younger and older mothers and between primiparae and multiparae, while there are apparently no such clear differences at age 10. Third, not only were we able to show important socio-cultural differences between the LBW and controls, even though they were matched for social class, but also impairments at age 10 seem to be differentiated according to social class.

Analytic strategy

The purpose of this analysis is to reveal which of the factors discussed above have an absolute and/or relative influence on the observed differences between the LBW children and the matched control group at 10 years old. There are two ways of answering this question. The first is to account for the actual outcomes observed amongst LBW children; while our study provides important evidence in this regard, it cannot be regarded as definitive because of the small number of cases involved. The second is to analyse the differences observed between the outcomes for LBW and control children.

It seems clear that the *actual* outcomes amongst LBW children should depend upon the *absolute* value of the variables observed at birth, although it might be argued that small initial *differences* between the LBW and control babies in the independent variables could eventually have a large effect upon the outcome for LBW children through a process of deviance amplification. The situation, however, is not so clear with the differences in outcome: these might depend upon the other differences observed between the LBW and control children or upon the absolute values observed for the LBW children. For example, the LBW children may be impaired because they are all *comparatively* lighter than their controls at birth or because their birthweight is, in *absolute terms*, low. The observed differences between the LBW and their controls in outcome scores (henceforth referred to as the observed impairment score) must, therefore, be analysed in terms both of the *differences* between the LBW and controls in respect of the variables studied at birth and of the absolute values for the same variables of the LBW children only.

Our major problem is the large number of variables, given that there are only about 140 LBW children. Indeed, one of the reasons for the analysis in Chapter 4 was to reduce the number of variables which needed to be considered in that chapter. For a similar reason the ordinal position of the child has been discarded due to its high correlation with parity. Even so, we still have too many potential variables since not only the absolute values have to be considered but the *differences* as well. To reduce the number of variables to be included we have proceeded as follows.

The first set of regressions analyses the outcome for the LBW children in terms of the actual values of the variables which are assumed to be important for development. Clearly, if a variable is important absolutely in determining the outcome for LBW children, it is also likely to be important relatively. A similar set of analyses was conducted for the control children and analogously, although this is affirmed with less conviction, a variable which is absolutely important for the control children might also be important relatively for LBW children. Note, however, that these latter analyses (for the control group) have not been discussed separately because the control group is *not* representative of a population of children of all birth weights (see Chapter 3) and because the important influences on the subsequent growth and mental development of 'normal' infants are better documented elsewhere (see, for example, Davie *et al.*, 1972).

The second step is the construction of difference scales *only* for those variables which appeared as *independently* influencing the outcome for either the LBW or the *control* groups. In most cases this has been done by subtraction of the values observed separately for the LBW and control children. However, the procedure was more complex for the sociological variables because they were indices which had been constructed for each of the identifiably distinct areas of sociological importance.

The second set of regressions analyse the impairment of LBW children relative to the controls and is therefore based upon the variables which have been found to have an independent absolute effect for the LBW group and upon the difference scales as constructed above. From these analyses the *main equations* which form the basis of our discussion were derived. However, at first sight many of the results are confusing or (apparently) contradictory or are opposite of what might be expected. Such results call for further analysis.

In particular, there might be sub-groups within the population in which the forms of the relationships are very different. A formal statistical test of this possibility can be conducted via the Chow test, wherein the same model (i.e. including the same variables) is estimated on the whole population and on the two sub-populations, and the reduction in the indical sums of squares is tested with an F statistic (see Hanushek and Jackson, 1977).

In this study each of the matching variables suggests a possible dichotomous or extreme sub-group of mothers for analysis, such as, for example, Social Classes I/V, smokers/non-smokers, mothers of male/female babies, primiparae/multiparae, and tall/short mothers. Empirically, we have already remarked upon the importance of maternal age in Chapter 4, with the proposal that younger and older mothers should be considered differently, which also suggests a separate analysis. One might also want to distinguish between growth-retarded and premature babies.

In fact, we have concentrated on possible differences between younger and older mothers and between growth-retarded and premature babies (groups 2 plus 4 and groups 1 plus 3, respectively, as defined in Chapter 5, page 95), that is, one division according to a characteristic of the mother and one division according to a characteristic of the baby. We note that, even so, there is some association between the two characteristics: thus of the 47 prematures, 32 mothers were under 25 and 15 were 25 or over; while of the 76 growth-retarded, 40 mothers were under 25 and 36 were 25 or over: however, this association does not reach statistical significance ($\chi^2 = 2.87$, $p = 0.08$).

THE SEPARATE ANALYSIS OF LBW AND CONTROL GROUPS

The detailed and full analysis of the determinants of intellectual and physical development among LBW children is long and complex. Because this detail is unlikely to interest the majority of our readers, a condensed summary of the results is presented at the beginning of each of the sections, leaving the detailed analysis to be included in small type.

An initial trial was performed aimed at reducing the number of variables by conducting *separate* regressions for the LBW and control groups of each of the eight outcome scores (full IQ, verbal IQ, performance IQ, Bender score, integration error score, height, weight and head circumference) on each of the four groups of independent variables. A liberal criterion of 20 per cent significance of the coefficient was used in each of these 64 regressions to determine which variables should be chosen for further analysis. Table 9.2 lists the variables which passed this hurdle for the LBW and control groups.

The next step of the regression analysis consists of combining the variables which have been selected on the basis of the four separate previous runs into one set of independent variables for each outcome variable, again treating the LBW and control groups separately. The eight outcome variables are considered in the three groups of 'mental', 'psycho-motor' and 'physical' development (see page 208).

The individual results for the regression analysis of the Bender scores do not add a great deal to what can be said on the basis of the regressions for the mental measurements. In the first place, there are very few coefficients which are significant, which suggests that on the whole the factors which influence psycho-motor development are not captured by the variables that we have measured in this study. Moreover, nearly all of the results that would otherwise be interesting in the regression analyses for the mental measurements include factors which positively influence IQ with a significant coefficient and also negatively influence the number of Bender errors. Therefore we have not presented a separate discussion for the Bender scores. However, when we come to assess the contributions of the different groups of variables we have included the results for the Bender scores for comparison (see Tables 9.7 and 9.13).

Variables selected in the fashion described above from each of the four groups in Table 9.1 were entered into combined regression equations, the selection being different, of course, for each of the eight outcome variables and for the various sub-populations (mothers under 25 and mothers 25 and over: growth-retarded and premature infants).

The results obtained when these selections are combined into a single regression equation are summarized in Tables 9.3 and 9.4 for the mental development and for the physical characteristics respectively for the whole population and for each of the sub-populations. As explained previously (page 212) the results are reported at or around the step at which the R^2 change falls below 2 per cent.

Measurement of mental (intellectual) development

Table 9.5 summarizes the results for the factors affecting intellectual development in LBW children. It can be seen that no variable appears significantly in all the sub-populations but several appear in more than one:

1. Maternal height appears negatively in the equation for the whole population and for growth retarded babies.
2. Parity appears negatively in the equation for older mothers, yet positively in the equation for premature babies.
3. Birth weight appears positively in the equation for the whole population and in the equations both for growth retarded and for premature babies.
4. Attitude to behaviour training appears negatively in every equation except the one for older mothers.
5. The interviewer's assessment appears positively in the equations for the whole population, for older mothers and for growth retarded babies.

Correlations

There is considerable overlap between the three IQ scales for the whole group: in particular, the independent variables which have the highest correlation coefficient with each of the scales tend to be the same. The three coefficients (in the order Full IQ, Verbal IQ, Performance IQ) for the six correlation coefficients which are the highest for the Full IQ scale are as follows:

1. Interviewer's assessment ($r = 0.33, 0.32, 0.25$). The higher the assessment of the mother, the higher the child's IQ:
2. Parental attitudes to behaviour training ($r = -0.24, -0.23, -0.23$). The more permissive the parents, the higher the child's IQ.

Table 9.2 Variables which entered significantly at the 20 per cent level in the separate equations for low birth weight (L) and control (C) children: (a) for intellectual development; (b) for physical development

(a)	All mothers			<25 years			≥25 years			Growth-retarded			Premature		
	FIQ	VIQ	PIQ	FIQ	VIQ	PIQ	FIQ	VIQ	PIQ	FIQ	VIQ	PIQ	FIQ	VIQ	PIQ
Matching															
Sex						L	L	L					L	L	
Social class		C					C	C		C	C				
Smoking	L	L	C	C	C		C	C		C	C	L			C
Maternal height	C	C	C	C	C	L	L	L		L	L	L	L	L	C
Parity	C	C													C
Neonatal															
Neo. problems	C	C		C	C	C	C	C	C	C	C	C	C	C	C
Gestational age	L	L	L	L	L	L	C	C	L	L	L		C	C	C
Days in SCBU									L						
Birth weight	L	L	L	L	L	L	L	L		L	L		L	L	L
Gen nutrit. state	C			L	L	L				L					
Maternal															
Del. complic.	C	C	L	C	C		C	C		C	C	L	C		C
Med. cond. of preg.			L												C
Med. compl. of preg.							C	C	C						C
Past obstet. history				L	L	L	C	C							
No. abortions				L	L	L	C	C						C	
Social															
Maternal age	L	L	L	C	L	C	L	C	L	L	L	L	C	C	C
Socio-cultural	C	C	C	L	L	C	C	C		C	L	C	L	L	L
Recreation activities			C						L						
Exp. to influence									C	C	C	C			
Behav. training	L	L	L	L	L	L	C	C		L	L		L	L	L
Husband's role	C	C					L	L							L
Maternal role							L	L							
Interviewer's assess.	L	L	L	C	C	C	L	L	L	L	L	L	C	C	C

(b)

	All mothers			<25 years			≥25 years			Growth retarded			Premature		
	Head circ.	Wt.	Ht.	Head circ.	Wt.	Ht.	Head circ.	Wt.	Ht.	Head circ.	Wt.	Ht.	Head circ.	Wt.	Ht.
Matching															
Sex	L	L					C	L			L	L	L		
Social class			L			L	L	L	L			L	L		
Smoking	C	C	L				C	C		L	C	C			C
Maternal height			C		C	L	C	C	L	L	C	C	C	C	L
Parity					C	C	C			C					
Neonatal															
Neo. problems	C	L		L	L	L	C	L		L			C	L	L
Gestational age	L	L	L	L	L	L	L			L			C	C	L
Days in SCBU	L	L	L	L	L	L	L			C	C		L	L	L
Birth weight	L	L	L	L	L	L	C	L		C	C	C	L	L	L
Gen. nutrit. state	C	L	L	C	L	L	C	L		C		C	C	C	C
Maternal															
Del. complic.	C	L		C			L	L	L	C			C		C
Med. cond. of preg.				C	L			L	C	C	C		C	C	
Med. compl. of preg.				L	L			C	C		L		C	L	
Past obstet. history													L	L	C
No. abortions		L		L	L										
Social															
Maternal age	C	C	C		L	L	L	L		C			C	L	L
Socio-cultural		C					L	L	C	C			C	C	
Recreation act.						C									L
Exp. to influence			C					L	C						
Behav. training	C	C	C		L		C	C	C		C	C	C	C	
Husband's role		C		L			C	L		L	C		C		
Maternal role	L	L	C	L	C				C	L		C		C	C
Interviewer's assess.	L	L	C	L			C	L	L	L		L	L		

Table 9.3   The values of the significant coefficients (together with their standard errors and t values) which enter the equations for intellectual development for LBW children

		Sex	Social class	Matching		Parity	Neonatal problems	Gest. age	Neonatal Days in SCBU	Birth weight	Gen. nutrit. state
				Smoking	Mat. height						
All mothers											
Full IQ	Coeff.	—	—	—	−0.604	—	—	−0.194	—	0.019	—
	S.E.				(0.285)			(0.114)		(0.008)	
	t				2.121			1.704		2.331	
Verbal IQ	Coeff.	—	—	—	−0.457	—	—	−0.217	—	0.019	—
	S.E.				(0.291)			(0.117)		(0.008)	
	t				1.572			1.865		2.318	
Perf. IQ	Coeff.	—	—	—	−0.712	—	—	−0.209	—	0.017	—
	S.E.				(0.284)			(0.115)		(0.008)	
	t				2.507			1.809		2.119	
Mothers <25											
Full IQ	Coeff.	—	—	—	—	—	—	—	—	—	4.423
	S.E.										(3.284)
	t										1.347
Verbal IQ	Coeff.	—	—	—	—	—	—	—	—	—	4.881
	S.E.										(3.335)
	t										1.462
Perf. IQ	Coeff.	−12.761	—	—	—	—	—	—	—	—	4.247
	S.E.	(5.12)									(3.09)
	t	2.494									1.375
Mothers ≥25											
Full IQ	Coeff.	−6.074	4.795	—	—	−2.323	—	—	−0.200	—	—
	S.E.	(3.316)	(4.639)			(1.283)			(−0.101)		
	t	1.832	1.034			1.811			1.985		
Verbal IQ	Coeff.	−6.859	—	—	—	—	—	—	−0.233	—	—
	S.E.	(3.372)							(0.098)		
	t	2.034							2.390		
Perf. IQ	Coeff.	—	—	—	—	−4.289	—	0.146	—	—	—
	S.E.					(1.224)		(0.087)			
	t					3.504		1.670			

Table 9.3 cont'd

		Mat. del complic.	Med. cond. of preg.	Pregnancy Med. complic.	Prev. Ob. hist	No. Abortions	Mat. age	Soc.-cul. env.	Recr. Act.	Exp. to Influ.	Att. to Behav. tr.	Social Husb. role	Mat. role	Inter. assess
All mothers														
Full IQ	Coeff.	—	—	—	—	—	0.749	—	—	—	−1.441	—	—	1.135
	S.E.						(0.299)				(0.769)			(0.330)
	t						2.505				1.873			3.440
Verbal IQ	Coeff.	—	—	—	—	—	0.749	—	—	—	−1.410	—	—	1.084
	S.E.						(0.306)				(0.786)			(0.337)
	t						2.444				1.794			3.216
Perf. IQ	Coeff.	—	−3.700	—	—	—	0.693	—	—	—	−1.200	—	—	0.918
	S.E.		(2.367)				(0.303)				(0.776)			(0.330)
	t		1.563				2.291				1.546			2.782
Mothers <25														
Full IQ	Coeff.	—	—	—	—	−17.503	—	1.764	—	—	−2.164	—	—	—
	S.E.					(7.500)		(1.142)			(1.104)			
	t					2.334		1.545			1.959			
Verbal IQ	Coeff.	—	—	—	—	−18.13	—	2.298	—	—	−1.765	—	—	—
	S.E.					(7.610)		(1.160)			(1.121)			
	t					1.981		1.981			1.574			
Perf. IQ	Coeff.	—	—	—	—	−15.975	—	1.981	—	—	−2.498	—	—	—
	S.E.					(6.840)					(1.034)			
	t					2.336					2.420			
Mothers ⩾25														
Full IQ	Coeff.	—	—	—	—	—	0.785	—	—	—	—	—	2.100	0.704
	S.E.						(0.461)						(2.225)	(0.356)
	t						1.703						0.944	1.977
Verbal IQ	Coeff.	—	—	—	—	—	—	—	—	—	—	—	3.611	0.908
	S.E.												(2.049)	(0.318)
	t												1.762	2.851
Perf. IQ	Coeff.	—	—	—	—	—	0.984	—	—	—	—	—	—	0.530
	S.E.						(0.465)							(0.306)
	t						2.117							1.731

Table 9.3 cont'd.

		Sex	Social class	Matching Smoking	Matching Mat. height	Parity	Neonatal problems	Gest. Age	Neonatal Days in SCBU	Neonatal Birth weight	Gen Nutrit. state
Growth-retarded											
Full IQ	Coeff.	—	—	—	-1.039	—	—	—	—	0.017	—
	S.E.				(0.390)					(0.011)	
	t				2.663					1.555	
Verbal IQ	Coeff.	—	—	—	-0.849	—	—	—	—	0.021	—
	S.E.				(0.390)					(0.011)	
	t				2.175					1.909	
Perf. IQ	Coeff.	—	—	—	-1.260	—	—	—	—	—	—
	S.E.				(0.398)						
	t				3.166						
Prematures											
Full IQ	Coeff.	—	12.296	—	—	6.121	—	—	—	0.012	—
	S.E.		(7.380)			(2.444)				(0.006)	
	t		1.666			2.504				1.912	
Verbal IQ	Coeff.	—	16.717	—	—	6.666	—	—	—	0.011	—
	S.E.		(7.611)			(2.521)				(0.006)	
	t		2.196			2.644				1.747	
Perf. IQ	Coeff.	—	—	—	—	—	—	—	—	0.011	—
	S.E.									(0.006)	
	t									1.788	

		Mat. del. complic.	Med. cond.	Pregnancy Med. complic.	Pregnancy Prev. ob. hist	No. of abortions	Mat age	Soc.-cul. env.	Recr. act.	Exp. to influ.	Att. to Behav. tr.	Social Husb. role	Mat. role	Inter. Assess.
Growth retarded														
Full IQ	Coeff.	—	—	—	—	—	0.762	—	—	—	-1.615	—	—	1.142
	S.E.						(0.382)				1.069			(0.435)
	t						1.994				1.512			2.621
Verbal IQ	Coeff.	—	—	—	—	—	0.569	2.271	—	—	-1.726	—	—	—
	S.E.						(0.401)	(0.899)			(1.075)			
	t						1.419	2.524			1.609			
Perf IQ	Coeff.	—	—	—	—	—	0.677	—	—	—	—	—	—	1.185
	S.E.						(0.394)							(0.429)
	t						1.719							2.760
Prematures														
Full IQ	Coeff.	—	—	—	—	—	—	—	—	—	-3.332	—	—	—
	S.E.										(1.156)			
	t										2.883			
Verbal IQ	Coeff.	—	—	—	—	—	—	—	—	—	-3.137	—	—	—
	S.E.										(1.192)			
	t								1.366		2.631			
Perf IQ	Coeff.										-2.555			

Table 9.4 The values of the significant coefficients (together with their standard errors and *t* values) which enter the equations for physical development for LBW children

		Sex	Social class	Matching Smoking	Mat. height	Parity	Neonatal problems	Gest. age	Days in SCBU	Neonatal Birth weight	Gen nutrit. state
All mothers											
Head cir.	Coeff.	-4.957	—	—	—	—	—	-0.207	—	0.017	—
	S.E.	(2.883)						(0.098)		(0.007)	
	t	1.719						2.11		2.636	
Weight	Coeff.	—	—	—	—	—	—	-0.521	-0.558	0.031	—
	S.E.							(0.312)	(0.208)	(0.021)	
	t							1.671	2.678	1.469	
Height	Coeff.	—	—	8.418	1.133	—	—	-0.283	—	0.025	-4.69
	S.E.			(4.303)	(0.335)			(0.150)		(0.010)	(2.93)
	t			1.956	3.378			1.889		2.372	1.59
Mothers <25											
Head cir.	Coeff.	—	—	—	—	—	—	—	—	0.009	—
	S.E.									(0.007)	
	t									1.388	
Weight	Coeff.	—	—	—	—	—	—	-0.503	-0.613	0.052	—
	S.E.							(0.358)	(0.282)	(0.025)	
	t							1.406	2.172	2.095	
Height	Coeff.	—	—	—	1.197	—	—	-0.480	—	0.041	-7.821
	S.E.				(0.390)			(0.174)		(0.012)	(3.662)
	t				3.072			2.748		3.472	2.132
Mothers ≥25											
Head cir.	Coeff.	—	—	-8.609	—	—	—	-0.306	-0.426	—	—
	S.E.			(3.649)				(0.146)	(0.176)		
	t			2.359				2.095	2.145		
Weight	Coeff.	18.597	—	—	—	—	-5.117	—	—	—	—
	S.E.	(11.198)					(3.500)				
	t	1.661					1.462				
Height	Coeff.	—	—	13.560	0.854	—	—	—	—	—	—
	S.E.			(7.22)	(0.587)						
	t			1.878	1.454						

Table 9.4 cont'd

		Mat del. complic.	Med. cond.	Pregnancy Med. complic.	Prev. ob. hist.	No. abortions	Mat. age	Soc.-cul. env.	Recr. act.	Exp. to influ.	Social Att to behav. tr.	Husb. role	Mat. role	Inter. assess.
All mothers														
Head cir.	Coeff.	—	—	—	—	—	—	—	—	—	—	—	—	2.415
	S.E.													(1.573)
	t													1.536
Weight	Coeff.	—	9.773	6.217	—	—	—	—	—	—	—	—	—	7.584
	S.E.		(5.848)	(6.100)										(4.740)
	t		1.671	1.02										1.600
Height	Coeff.	—	—	—	—	—	—	—	—	—	—	—	—	—
	S.E.													
	t													
Mothers <25														
Head cir.	Coeff.	—	—	—	—	−12.817	—	—	—	—	—	—	−1.319	0.949
	S.E.					(5.385)							(0.898)	(0.477)
	t					2.38							1.469	1.990
Weight	Coeff.	—	—	—	33.237	−53.868	—	—	—	—	—	—	—	—
	S.E.				(23.169)	(27.208)								
	t				1.435	1.98								
Height	Coeff.	—	—	—	—	—	—	—	—	—	—	—	—	—
	S.E.													
	t													
Mothers ≥25														
Head cir.	Coeff.	6.292	—	—	—	—	—	—	—	—	—	—	—	—
	S.E.	(1.776)												
	t	3.543												
Weight	Coeff.	11.654	14.148	—	—	—	—	—	—	—	—	—	5.789	—
	S.E.	(5.608)	(6.142)										(2.071)	
	t	2.078	2.303										2.794	
Height	Coeff.	—	—	—	—	—	—	—	—	—	—	—	—	0.824
	S.E.													(0.596)
	t													1/383

		Sex	Social class	Matching Smoking	Matching Mat. height	Parity	Neonatal problems	Gest. age	Days in SCBU	Neonatal Birth weight	Gen. nutrit. state
Growth retarded											
Head Cir.	Coeff.	—	—	—	−0.805	—	—	−0.475	—	0.018	—
	S.E.				(0.311)			(0.190)		(0.009)	
	t				2.586			2.498		1.951	
Weight	Coeff.	25.815	—	9.610	—	—	—	—	−0.651	—	—
	S.E.	(10.319)		(5.790)					(0.262)		
	t	2.502		1.66					2.485		
Height	Coeff.	8.826	—	—	—	—	—	—	—	—	—
	S.E.	(4.999)									
	t	1.766									
Prematures											
Head Cir.	Coeff.	−8.931	—	—	—	3.337	—	—	—	0.009	—
	S.E.	(4.954)				(1.794)				(0.006)	
	t	1.803				1.86				1.66	
Weight	Coeff.	—	—	—	—	—	—	—	—	0.026	—
	S.E.									(0.016)	
	t									1.584	
Height	Coeff.	—	—	—	2.605	—	—	—	—	0.019	—
	S.E.				(0.456)					(0.007)	
	t				5.716					2.685	

		Mat. del complic.	Med. cond.	Pregnancy Med. complic.	Prev. ob. hist.	No. of abortions	Mat. age	Soc.-cul. env.	Recr. Act.	Exp. to influ.	Social Att. to Behav. tr.	Husb. role	Mat. role	Inter. assess.
Growth retarded														
Head cir	Coeff.	—	—	—	—	—	—	—	—	—	—	—	5.727	—
	S.E.												(2.105)	
	t												2.721	
Weight	Coeff.	—	—	14.987	—	—	—	—	—	—	—	—	—	—
	S.E.			(6.349)										
	t			2.361										
Height	Coeff.	—	—	—	—	—	—	—	—	—	—	—	—	0.700
	S.E.													(0.475)
	t													1.473
Premature														
Head Cir.	Coeff.	—	—	—	—	−2.821	—	—	—	—	—	—	—	0.686
	S.E.					(2.352)								(0.499)
	t					1.199								1.374
Weight	Coeff.	—	—	—	37.319	−46.704	2.878	—	—	—	—	—	—	—
	S.E.				(20.005)	(1.298)	(1.298)							
	t				1.865	2.101	2.217							
Height	Coeff.	—	—	—	—	—	1.038	—	2.521	—	—	—	—	—
	S.E.						(0.494)		(0.771)					
	t						2.101		3.269					

Table 9.5 Significant coefficients which appear in at least two of the equations for intellectual development

	Matching	Pregnancy	Neonatal	Social
All mothers	Maternal height (−)	—	Gestational age (−) Birth weight (+)	Att. to behav. training (−) Inter. assessment (+)
Younger mothers	—	No abortions (−)	—	Att. to behav. training (−) Soc.-cult. environment (+)
Older mothers	Sex (M) Parity (−)	—	Days in SCBU (−)	Maternal role (+) Int. assessment (+)
Growth retarded babies	Maternal height (−)	—	Birth weight (+)	Maternal age (+) Att. to behav. training (−) Int. assessment (+)
Premature babies	Social class (+) Parity (+)	—	Birth weight (+)	Att. to behav. training (−)

Notes 1. The entries in the table show which variables appeared with coefficients significant at the 20 per cent level in at least two of the three equations which were estimated for intellectual development.
2. A positive sign means that 'more of' the factor improves the outcome.

3. Socio-cultural environment ($r = 0.24, 0.27, 0.17$). The more diverse and educated the background, the higher the child's IQ.
4. Social class at matching ($r = 0.24, 0.25, 0.16$). Children of non-manual worker fathers tend to have higher IQ.
5. Mother's age ($r = 0.24, 0.23, 0.20$). Children of older mothers tend to have higher IQ scores.
6. Birth weight ($r = 0.21, 0.19, 0.20$). The greater a child's birth weight, the higher the IQ.

It is not surprising that the interviewers' assessments of the mothers' fluency, rationality, and vocabulary are highly correlated with the child's IQ. For, inasmuch as the interviewer made a correct assessment, these are precisely the qualities which are crucial in developing the child's intelligence within the mother–child relationship. Moreover, these qualities could be quite highly correlated with the mother's own intelligence. The next three variables all reflect different facets of social status, as permissiveness and a diverse cultural environment tend to be associated with families where the head of the household is in a non-manual occupation. Moreover, these three variables are all reasonably highly intercorrelated with each other and with the interviewer's assessment of them.

The other two variables have a different status. Thus, older mothers tend to have children of higher IQ and, since it is unlikely that ageing *per se* influences the offspring's IQ, this is probably an artefact of other relationships. Birth weight is the most important medically/biologically assessed variable to be correlated with IQ: whether or not this is a true effect or due to intervening social and/or medical variables will be evident from the regression analysis.

Regressions

For the whole population, six variables appear consistently and usually significantly in the equations. Thus the child's subsequent IQ is higher if the mother is shorter, if the baby was prematurely born, if the baby was heavier at birth, if the mother was older, if the mother had a more flexible attitude to behaviour training, and if the interviewer's assessment of the mother was more positive.

Most of these results are similar to what has been reported from other studies on the relationship between conditions at or around birth and subsequent intellectual development (see Chapter 2), and confirm the importance of socio-economic variables in influencing intellectual development. But the results for maternal height and gestational age at birth are, when taken in isolation, surprising, since other results show maternal height and gestational age to be positively related to IQ. We note, however, that the result for birth weight—which is, of course, positively associated with gestational age—goes in the expected direction. We can interpret these results provisionally as saying that it is more 'normal' and therefore less detrimental to subsequent outcome for a shorter mother to produce a LBW baby and/or for such a baby to be born prematurely. A breakdown of average IQ according to both height of mother and whether or not the LBW baby was growth-retarded or premature is suggestive. For while it shows no clear relationship between the height of the mother and the IQ of the child, there is a two point difference in the subsequent IQ between babies who were growth retarded and those who were premature, in favour of the latter. At the same time, among LBW babies, the heavier the baby the better the subsequent outcome.

Nevertheless, the finding prompts further analysis to explore the *form* of the relationship. We attempted a variety of analyses within different sub-groups. The most successful split was that between younger and older mothers and this was confirmed by the

Table 9.6 Residual sums of squares and F values of Chow tests for assessing best split of total populations when analysing absolute scores for LBW children

	Total population	Splitting by maternal age		Splitting by fetal growth	
		<25	≥25	Growth-retarded	Premature
Intellectual development	($n=115$)	($n=65$)	($n=50$)	($n=67$)	($n=37$)
(12 variables included)					
Full IQ	37102.7	24304.1	5445.1	24465.2	3610.6
F values		1.874		1.403	
Verbal IQ	38714.0	26550.7	5399.3	24634.4	4122.7
F values		1.605		1.618	
Performance IQ	35987.7	22205.9	6280.4	25262.9	3684.8
F values		1.997		1.056	
Physical development	($n=112$)	($n=65$)	($n=47$)	($n=67$)	($n=39$)
(14 variables included)					
Height	22756.9	13147.8	4237.1	12281.2	4964.0
F values		1.809		1.958	
Weight	201240.1	103619.8	44406.2	104881.4	37269.8
F values		2.106		2.500	
Head circum.	45250.4	20910.7	15758.5	24269.3	8890.5
F values		1.370		2.188	

Chow test as shown in Table 9.6. Thus, for the young mothers, the child's subsequent IQ is higher if the LBW baby appeared as her first pregnancy, rather than after one or more abortions; if the general nutritional status of the baby looked good; the more flexible the mother in her attitude to behaviour training; and the better the socio-cultural environment around birth. For older mothers, the child's subsequent IQ is higher if he is a boy; if he is the first child; the fewer the days spent in the special care baby unit; the older the mother; the greater her preparation for motherhood; and the higher the interviewer's assessment.

If the division in our sample is made according to the baby, i.e. whether the LBW child is premature or growth-retarded, a certain commonality of factors is noted. Birth weight, i.e. the heavier the child, and parental attitudes to behaviour training, i.e. more flexible attitudes, are found to be beneficial for both groups. We note also that gestational age does *not* enter either of these two sub-groups which presumably indicates that, among the whole population, gestational age surrogates for this split. Otherwise the equation for growth-retarded babies is identical to that for the whole population. However, for the premature group, higher social class and higher parity are also associated with favourable outcome—neither of these latter results is unexpected.

Discussion

The results are clearly different for younger and older mothers and both are different from the overall population, which supports our earlier arguments (see Chapter 4). We shall explore these differences, first, by looking at the relative contributions of the four groups of variables in the sub-populations to the variance in IQ at age 10 and, second, by looking at the patterns of variables which appear in the various sets of equations.

First, then, we consider Table 9.7 which compares the R^2 obtained at the maximum step in each of the four separate regressions with that obtained in the combined regression for each of the eight outcome scores and for the population and each of the sub-populations separately. Note that we are using these figures comparatively so that it is of little importance whether we use the unadjusted or adjusted R^2 so long as we are consistent.

The first comment is that each group of variables makes a distinct contribution in that, in every case, the R^2 for the combined selected variables is much larger than the R^2 for the separate equations.

In considering the three IQ measurements, Table 9.7 shows that the sociological variables made the largest contribution in predicting outcome for the whole population. This suggests that the determination of IQ among LBW children depends mostly on socio-cultural features of their upbringing, although among older mothers basic features such as sex and parity are also important while among younger mothers the conditions around the pregnancy and delivery are relatively more important.

Second, the regressions presented in Table 9.3 have shown that completely different sets of variables appear for younger and older mothers, and are different from those for the whole population. Thus, the combination of variables which appeared in the whole population (maternal height, gestational age, birthweight, maternal age, attitudes to behaviour training, and interviewer's assessment) highlights the 'normality' of LBW among short mothers and premature babies.

On the other hand, for younger mothers the variables which are important (the number of abortions, general nutritional status, socio-cultural environment and parental attitudes to behaviour training) highlight the potential for good reproductive efficiency counteracting social deprivation; while for older mothers, the important variables (sex of infant and parity, number of days spent in special care baby unit, the extent of maternal role preparation and the interviewer's assessment of the mother) are more related to a healthy baby coupled with the articulate, experienced mother's commitment to pregnancy and a specific family structure.

Physical characteristics: absolute values

Table 9.8 summarizes the results for the factors affecting physical development among LBW children. Only three variables appear significantly in more than one equation:

1. Gestational age appears negatively in the equations for the whole population and for younger mothers;
2. Birth weight appears positively in the equation for the whole population, for younger mothers and for premature babies;
3. The number of abortions appears negatively in the equations for younger mothers and for premature babies.

Correlations

Although not to the same extent as with the mental measurement, there is an overlap between the sets of variables which separately have high simple correlations with actual head circumference, actual weight, and actual height. Therefore, we shall report the triad of coefficients (height, weight, head circumference), putting aside, for the moment, the high (genetic) correlation of maternal height with child's actual height (0.34).

Table 9.7 The contribution of different groups of variables to the prediction of absolute values for LBW children

	Full IQ	Verbal IQ	Perf. IQ	Bender Gestalt	Bender Integ.	Head circum.	Weight	Height
All mothers								
All	26.7	24.6	24.1	15.0	11.8	15.1	16.2	25.9
Matching	7.7	7.9	4.8	3.4	1.7	2.8	2.9	18.0
Neonatal	7.6	7.8	7.5	9.3	11.1	5.8	7.2	6.3
Preg.	1.4	1.2	1.8	0.8	0.9	5.7	4.7	5.6
Sociolog.	13.9	13.2	11.1	9.9	0.4	6.4	4.9	11.4
Mothers under 25								
All	24.1	22.7	28.4	23.4	12.4	24.2	27.2	41.7
Matching	3.1	3.0	4.2	3.7	5.0	2.6	1.3	21.5
Neonatal	10.3	10.2	10.3	9.7	14.9	9.2	10.9	24.7
Preg.	13.6	12.0	15.1	7.6	4.3	14.2	9.6	10.1
Sociolog.	11.0	10.0	12.0	17.0	3.7	13.9	4.7	11.8
Mothers over 25								
All	51.7	46.2	45.5	21.9	31.4	34.1	47.9	41.4
Matching	26.7	22.9	25.7	9.7	7.8	6.7	7.9	21.0
Neonatal	13.0	11.1	11.3	7.0	8.0	7.9	6.6	3.1
Preg.	15.9	9.3	22.7	8.1	12.3	16.5	19.9	4.8
Sociolog.	34.9	30.2	30.2	12.8	10.6	9.0	19.3	10.7
Growth-retarded babies								
All	32.9	32.9	27.8	35.4	32.5	41.3	32.8	28.4
Matching	13.4	10.8	13.3	11.3	8.8	4.7	5.5	14.2
Neonatal	9.4	8.7	10.2	9.1	15.9	8.3	10.3	4.5
Preg.	2.7	1.5	4.2	8.5	1.9	5.7	28.6	4.9
Sociolog.	18.8	18.4	14.8	13.2	3.3	3.8	2.8	10.1
Premature babies								
All	48.0	36.5	40.1	35.8	41.9	55.7	53.6	59.1
Matching	11.1	14.1	6.5	15.5	14.2	19.9	4.9	27.4
Neonatal	11.0	10.5	9.7	20.5	23.9	15.9	13.4	21.0
Preg.	7.5	6.7	5.6	12.9	10.1	11.8	13.0	11.4
Sociolog.	20.2	19.4	19.9	8.0	12.1	9.4	5.2	14.5

Table 9.8   Significant coefficients which appear in at least two of the equations for physical development

	Matching	Pregnancy	Neonatal	Social
All others	—	—	Gestational age (−) Birth weight (+)	Maternal role prep. (+)
Younger others	—	No. abortions (−)	Gestational age (−) Birth weight (+)	—
Older others	—	Maternal deliv. complic. (+)	—	—
Growth-retarded babies	Sex (F)	—	—	—
Premature babies	—	No. abortions (−)	Birth weight (+)	Maternal age (+)

Notes 1. The entries in the table show which variables appeared with coefficients significant at the 20 per cent level in at least two of the three equations which were estimated for physical development.
2. A positive sign means that 'more of' the factor improves the outcome.

1. Interviewer's assessments ($r = 0.25, 0.04, 0.13$), the higher the assessment, the bigger the child.
2. Number of previous abortions ($r = 0.19, 0.19, 0.07$), the greater the number, the bigger the child.
3. Socio-cultural environment ($r = 0.17, 0.19, 0.11$), the more diverse and educated the parents, the bigger the child.
4. Maternal role preparation ($r = 0.15, 0.14, 0.17$), the more formal preparation by the mother, the bigger the child.
5. Medical conditions specific to pregnancies ($r = 0.19, 0.19, 0.07$), the more conditions, the bigger the child.
6. Birth weight ($r = 0.07, 0.18, 0.15$), the bigger the baby, the bigger the child.

Of these six correlations we note first that the child's physical development is associated with physiological characteristics of the pregnancy and of the birth. Thus, a mother who has had a previous abortion will have a bigger child and, as the correlations with birth weight show, this is related to subsequent physical development. The same is true for most of the medical conditions specific to pregnancies. The first, third, and fourth correlations listed above, however, all support the contention that physical development also depends on social features which appear to operate within social class: the more favourable the interviewer's assessment, the 'better' the socio-cultural environment, the better prepared the mother, the larger the child.

Regressions

For the whole population, where five variables appear in the equation for actual height, seven for actual weight, and four in the equation for actual head circumference, there are four variables which appear in two or more of the equations. Thus, among matching variables the sex of the infant is related to both head circumference and weight, while present height is positively affected by maternal height and non-smoking.

Second, among the neonatal variables, gestational age has a negative effect while birth weight has a positive effect on all three developmental characteristics. This is similar to the finding for mental measurements and can be similarly explained. And, once again, none of the pregnancy variables appear to consistently influence physical outcome.

Finally, amongst the sociological variables, the only variable which appears consistently is maternal role preparation, where mothers who have been to classes, etc., have children with larger heads and bodies.

Once again, the results prompted us to attempt more detailed analysis. The most successful was the split between growth-retarded and premature children and this was confirmed by the Chow test (see Table 9.6). For, although we find very few consistent effects for growth-retarded children, there are three coefficients which appear in at least two of the equations for premature babies. Thus the child's subsequent physical development is greater if the baby was not preceded by one or more abortions, if the baby was heavier and the mother older at delivery. Other variables only appear in single equations: we note that the influence of maternal height on child's subsequent height remains for premature but not for growth-retarded babies, which is understandable: but the other once-only coefficients have no similar rationale.

Discussion

It is evident that, unlike mental measurements, there are few consistent patterns within the sub-groups for physical development. This would tend to indicate that this study has failed to capture the relevant important variables. Moreover, the significance of a large head or a heavy child, unlike height, is debatable and perhaps it is more the proportions than actual measurements which are important.

Table 9.7 shows the relative contribution of each group of variables to the physical outcome scores. It is apparent that, for height, the group of matching variables (which includes maternal height) makes the largest contribution overall and also within each sub-group, with the marginal exception that in younger mothers the contribution of neonatal factors is slightly greater. No similar consistency appears for weight or head circumference though in the former case pregnancy and neonatal factors tend to predominate.

Next, we examine the combination of variables which appear in the separate equation for the different sub-groups (Table 9.4). First we note that the most consistent finding is the positive association of maternal and child height with the exception of the growth retarded sub-group. Next, we see that not only is maternal age rarely significant but the pattern of significant coefficients does not vary systematically as between the separately estimated equations.

Indeed, more can be learnt from the split between growth-retarded and premature babies. Thus, the fact that we cannot find consistent relationships between the subsequent physical development of growth-retarded babies and any of the independent factors—including maternal height—means that the negative effect of growth retardation on subsequent physical development is not mediated by any of the factors taken into account in this analysis. Given that growth retardation as a condition is associated with specific physiological characteristics of pregnancy, this is hardly surprising. Although we checked to see if we could explicate the apparent relationship between growth retardation and maternal height via medical complication of pregnancy or maternal delivery complications no obvious relationship emerged.

On the other hand, our analysis suggests that the effects of premature birth can be mitigated if the baby is heavier (within the LBW range), if the baby is born to an older mother and/or if the mother has not previously had an abortion. The first factor is obvious, the second is consistent with the fact that premature birth to an older mother who has a good reproductive history is no significant disadvantage.

THE RELATIVE SIGNIFICANCE OF LOW BIRTH WEIGHT

A summary of the results is included in Tables 9.9 and 9.10 for intellectual and physical impairment respectively. Especial caution should be exercised in reading these tables as variables have been excluded when both the absolute value and the difference value for the same variable appeared in the same equation but with (effectively) equal and opposite signs.

Three sets of variables were included in the regression runs to determine LBW children's impairment. First, from the regression runs which described the factors affecting LBW outcome, we selected those variables which were found to be significant at the 20 per cent level. Second, difference scales for each of these variables were constructed by subtracting the absolute values observed for the LBW child from that observed for their control. In addition, the difference scale of any variable found to be significant in the comparable control regression runs which did not appear in the LBW population was also included (see Analytic Strategy p. 216, for rationale). These extra variables are indicated with a 'C' in Table 9.2. Thus those variables derived from the LBW population (L) will include their absolute and difference scale while the additional variables from the control population (C) will only include the difference scale.

The purpose of this part of the analysis is twofold: first, to provide supplementary evidence as to the factors which influence the poorer neurological, perceptuo-motor, and physical outcomes; and second, to assess whether it is the imbalance *between* the LBW baby and its control at birth or, alternatively, the varying experiences within the LBW group which are most important in affecting outcome.

Once again a variable is significant when the coefficient is significant at the 5 per cent level or better and the results reported are those at or around the step in the stepwise regression when the change in R^2 is below 2 per cent.

The mean and standard deviation of the impairment on the eight outcome scores are reported in Table 9.11. It can be seen that, although the average impairment is not very large, there is considerable variation to explain. This is important, in the first place, because it means that LBW does not *per se* have a very large influence on subsequent mental and physical development: in the second place, because it means that even when matched for variables which are known to be associated with subsequent development, such as parity, sex, social class, maternal height, and smoking, the relative impairment of a LBW child depends on a large number of other factors some of which may be amenable to social remedy.

As we explained in the first part of the chapter, the analysis of impairment will be in terms of both the absolute values for the LBW child and differences between the values observed for the LBW child and the corresponding control.

Table 9.9 Significant coefficients which appear in at least two of the equations for relative intellectual impairment

	Matching	Pregnancy	Neonatal	Social
All mothers	—	—	Diff. no. neo. prob. (−)	Diff. in mat. age (+) Int. ass. of LBW (+) Diff. in socio.-cult. env. (+) Att. to behav. training (+)
Younger mothers	Diff. in parity (+)	—	Diff. no. neo. prob. (−) Gestat. age (+)	Diff. in socio.-cult. env. (+) [Diff. in] att. to behav. training (+)
Older mothers	—	—	Diff. no. neo. prob. (−)	[Diff. in] mat. age (+/+)
Growth-retarded babies	Maternal height (−)	—	Diff. no. neo. prob. (−)	Diff. in mat. age (+) Diff. in socio.-cult. env. (+) Int. ass. of LBW (+)
Premature babies	Parity (+) Diff. in parity (+) Diff. in soc. class (−)	Diff. in no. mat. del. complic. (+)	Diff. no. neo. prob. (−)	Diff. in socio.-cult. env. (+)

Notes
1. The entries in the Table show which variables appeared with coefficients significant at the 20 per cent level in at least two of the three equations which were estimated for relative intellectual impairment.
2. A positive sign means that the less difference there is between the LBW case and the control in respect of the factor, the less relatively impaired is the LBW child relative to the control in intellectual development.
3. Where the absolute value of a variable appeared in one of the equations and the difference in another (but with the same sign), the factor has been included in the table using square brackets to indicate the situation.

Table 9.10 Significant coefficients which appear in at least two of the equations for relative physical impairment

	Matching	Pregnancy	Neonatal	Social
All mothers	—	—	Diff. in gen. nut. state (−)	—
Younger mothers	—	—	Diff. in birth weight (+) Diff. in gestat. age (−)	—
Older mothers	Diff. in maternal ht. (+)	No mat. del. complic. (+)	—	—
Growth retarded babies	—	—	Diff. in birth weight (+)	—
Premature babies	Diff. in maternal ht. (+)	Diff. in no. abort. (+)	Diff. in birth weight (+) Diff. in gen. nut. stat. (−)	Maternal age (+) Diff. in mat. role prep. (+)

Notes
1. The entries in the table show which variables appeared with coefficients significant at the 20 per cent level in at least two of the three equations which were estimated for relative physical impairment.
2. A positive sign means that the less difference there is between the LBW case and the control in respect of the factor, the less relatively impaired is the LBW child relative to the control in physical development.

Table 9.11   Mean and standard deviation of the impairment on the eight outcome scores

Impairment in	Scale	Mean	Standard deviation
Full IQ	50–150	−4.35	19.30
Verbal IQ	50–150	−2.64	19.49
Performance IQ	50–150	−4.39	19.50
Bender Gestalt	0–30	+0.66	2.82
Bender integration	0–9	+0.35	1.13
Actual head circum.	480–600 (in 0.1cm)	−5.44	22.18
Actual weight	200–500 (in 0.1kg)	−17.32	68.82
Actual height	250–600 (in 0.1in.)	−9.71	27.41

In reading the equations, it should be remembered that the difference scales of both the dependent and the independent variables have been constructed by subtracting the value for the control from the value for the LBW child. The difference scales for the outcome score will themselves be typically negative, and the values of these difference scales will tend to be negative for factors which we expect to improve outcome and tend to be positive for factors which we expect to worsen outcome. Regardless of the typical signs of the difference scales, we would expect positive coefficients for favourable factors and negative coefficients for unfavourable factors.

The influence on IQ impairment

The Summary Table 9.9 shows that the most consistent findings with respect to intellectual development relate to:

1. The difference in the number of neonatal problems which appears negatively in every equation.
2. The difference in socio-cultural environment which appears positively in every equation except the one for older mothers.

Only four other variables appear in more than one of the sub-populations:

3. The difference in parity, which appears positively in the equations for young mothers and for premature babies.
4. The difference in maternal age, which appears positively in the equations for the whole population, for the older mothers and for growth retarded babies.
5. The interviewer's assessment of the LBW mother which appears positively in the equations for the whole population and for growth retarded babies.

6. (Difference in) attitudes to behaviour training which appears positively in the equations for the whole population and for younger mothers.

We reiterate that this is a highly condensed summary of a quite detailed set of results which are explored more fully below.

Correlations

There is considerable overlap between the three IQ scales in terms of the sets of independent variables which have high correlations with the scales, therefore, they are reported as a triad (Full IQ, Verbal IQ, Performance IQ). The six highest are:

1. Differences in ages ($r = 0.29, 0.26, 0.26$), the younger the LBW mother relative to her control, the larger the IQ impairment.
2. Differences in interviewer's assessment ($r = 0.24, 0.20, 0.17$), the poorer the interviewer's assessment of the LBW mother relative to her control, the larger the IQ impairment.
3. Differences in neonatal problems index ($r = -0.23, -0.17, -0.22$), the more neonatal problems affecting the LBW child relative to the control, the larger the IQ impairment.
4. Birth weight ($r = 0.21, 0.17, 0.16$), the heavier the LBW child at birth (while, of course, being under 2500 g), the lower the IQ impairment.
5. Gestational age ($r = 0.21, 0.17, 0.16$), the greater the gestational age of the LBW child at birth, the lower the IQ impairment.
6. Maternal age ($r = 0.20, 0.18, 0.22$), the older the mother, the lower the IQ impairment.

We note also the relatively high correlation of full IQ impairment negatively with the differences between the parental recreational activities ($r = -0.19$), of verbal impairment positively with differences in parental socio-cultural environment ($r = 0.21$) and of performance IQ impairment positively with attitudes to behaviour training of LBW parents ($r = 0.18$) and negatively with the height of the LBW mother ($r = -0.19$) and differences between the parental recreational activities ($r = -0.19$).
difference in ages and the difference in interviewers' assessments) reflect social impairments. We note, too, that the absolute values of the same variables also had high correlation coefficients with the absolute IQ scores. Moreover, the relationship between the LBW mother's age relative to her control and IQ impairment is reinforced by the fact that the LBW mother's age itself also affects IQ impairment negatively. The two other correlation coefficients, between birth weight and gestational age and IQ impairment, go in the expected direction. In addition, we note that the correlations of the difference in neonatal problems are almost as high as for the two social difference variables and it will be interesting to see if this effect remains through the multivariate analysis.

Regressions

The first thing to note about the regression analysis is the pairing of coefficients of a variable with its corresponding difference scale. For example, both the general nutritional status of the LBW child and differences between the LBW and the control in general nutritional status enter the equations for full IQ impairment for mother under 25 (although not for the other sub-populations); but the coefficients are of opposite sign, so that a LBW child of lower *general nutritional status* than the average LBW child is associated with a larger IQ impairment while a LBW child who, relative to his control, is of poorer general nutritional status, is associated with a smaller IQ impairment. And, although the standardized betas (which measure the effect of a change of one standard deviation in each of the independent variables) are not equal (they are $+11.6$ and -7.8) their moduli are well within their standard errors. The same is true of *birth weight* of the LBW child and of differences in birth weight where the counter-intuitive result that a LBW child who is heavier than average has apparently a larger IQ impairment becomes clearer when seen in the context of the result that a LBW child who is relatively close in weight to his control has a smaller IQ impairment; and once again the standardized betas are of the same magnitude.

Similar pairings occur in the other equations. It is difficult to attach more importance to any such coefficients because of this complementarity.

In the total population, three factors emerged as affecting all three IQ impairment scores. Thus the LBW child is found to be less impaired the fewer the neonatal problems in comparison to his control, the older the LBW mother relative to her control, and the higher the interviewer's assessment of the LBW mother. In addition, socio-cultural factors were found to affect full and verbal IQ whereby the more advantaged the environment of the LBW child relative to the control, the less the subsequent impairment, and the more rigid the LBW mother's attitude to behaviour training, the less impairment there was found in the full and performance IQ scores.

If we compare the two maternal age groups, the importance of neonatal problems remains for both groups and the two socio-cultural factors for younger mothers. Also, the greater the parity of the LBW mother in relation to her control, the lower the noted impairment of the LBW child on full and performance IQ. For older mothers, impairment on full and verbal IQ is lower where the interviewer's assessment of the LBW mother is high. By splitting the whole population in this way, maternal age unsurprisingly fails to

Table 9.12 Residual sums of squares and F values of Chow tests for assessing best split of total populations when analysing impairments

	Total population	Splitting by maternal age		Splitting by fetal growth	
		<25	≥25	Growth-retarded	Premature
Intellectual development (18 variables included)	$(n=109)$	$(n=60)$	$(n=49)$	$(n=36)$	$(n=66)$
Full IQ	28077.2	12032.2	9856.6	5104.4	13400.3
	F values		1.147		2.098
Verbal IQ	30985.8	12660.9	10260.3	5823.1	13197.3
	F values		1.427		2.551
Performance IQ	27822.7	11883.5	98490.0	6587.1	13864.7
	F values		1.139		1.462
Physical development (14 variables included)	$(n=106)$	$(n=61)$	$(n=45)$	$(n=35)$	$(n=65)$
Height	57469.2	22108.4	27716.7	11387.6	32583.2
	F values		0.877		1.889
Weight	334963.8	185843.5	103927.3	81274.3	181731.6
	F values		0.981		1.707
Head circum.	34282.9	13426.6	10965.6	11138.0	15169.2
	F values		2.495		1.698

have importance, but otherwise the differences are minor (as confirmed by the Chow test results in Table 9.12).

If, however, we divide the LBW population into prematures and growth-retarded infants, different patterns emerge though both feature neonatal problems and socio-cultural factors (see Table 9.12 for Chow test). Within the growth-retarded group, mothers who were shorter, who were highly assessed by the interviewer, and who tended to be older than their controls, were found to have less impaired children. Once again the evidence suggests that when tall mothers have growth-retarded children there is something definitely wrong. For LBW prematures, the children of mothers with absolute higher parity and higher parity in relation to their controls, with more delivery complication, and of lower social class, tended to be less impaired. These results again indicate the concomitance of high parity and prematurity as being 'normal'. The finding that more delivery complications are beneficial probably reflects timely obstetric intervention.

Discussion

The pattern is relatively clear here and interestingly different from the pattern with the absolute values. The obvious difference is that an index of neonatal problems consistently appears in the equations for impairment and not at all in the equations for absolute values. We investigate the balance between the different groups of variables through their relative contributions to the variance and, once again, through the pattern of variables which appears in the equations.

Table 9.13 gives the contribution of the different groups of variables to the prediction of impairment for all the eight outcome variables. For the whole population we can see that the neonatal and sociological variables make a roughly equal contribution. However, when we consider the separate regressions for growth-retarded and premature babies, the balance shifts towards the sociological variables in the equations for impairment in full and for verbal IQ. The neonatal variables only predominate in the equation for younger mothers while in the other sub-populations the pregnancy variables become more important.

The pattern of the coefficients is different in the equations for growth-retarded and for premature babies and there are also interesting differences between these sub-populations and the overall population. They show that, although the neonatal problems index is nearly always significant, sociological variables also enter the equations but in different ways in the different sub-populations. One can typify the differences by saying that the sub-population of growth-retarded babies seems to be homogeneous in terms of the factors which affect subsequent intellectual development, while the sub-population of premature babies is such that the kind of impact upon later development depends upon what other factors are associated with the premature birth.

Another approach to this problem was to search for the variables which discriminate between those who are most impaired and those who are least impaired. To this end a discriminant function analysis was conducted in which the following two groups were defined: one, when the LBW child scores lower than the control in respect of *each* of the IQ variables; and the other, when the LBW child scores higher than the control in respect of *at least one* of the IQ variables.

The results are presented in Table 9.14. The first part of the Table shows that the group of 51 LBW children who perform uniformly worse than their controls have *much* lower average IQs (differences of 15.6, 15.6 and 12.2) and that they are much more homogeneous (the standard deviations are considerably lower).

The discriminant function analysis itself was performed stepwise so that we have presented the results in the order of their entry into the calculation of the discriminant

Table 9.13   The contribution of different groups of variables to the prediction of the impairment of LBW children

	Full IQ R^2	Verbal IQ R^2	Perf. IQ R^2	Bender Gestalt R^2	Bender Integ. R^2	Head Circum. R^2	Weight R^2	Height R^2
All mothers								
All	34.9	33.5	35.0	21.4	19.5	43.4	37.9	29.7
Matching	9.5	7.4	12.6	5.0	8.1	12.1	13.1	16.8
Neonatal	13.9	12.2	12.4	4.2	13.5	32.8	32.3	19.4
Preg.	4.6	5.3	6.1	7.2	3.3	9.5	8.7	10.8
Sociolog.	13.8	12.3	15.1	9.4	9.9	13.8	11.0	11.5
Mothers under 25								
All	36.4	52.3	40.3	19.8	14.8	58.8	42.9	45.1
Matching	7.9	6.4	12.5	10.7	11.0	9.2	10.1	17.6
Neonatal	23.4	21.8	17.3	9.5	24.6	45.5	44.2	40.3
Preg.	7.1	9.4	9.7	13.5	11.9	16.3	15.2	8.0
Sociolog.	20.9	21.5	23.9	15.1	18.2	24.8	22.9	19.8
Mothers over 25								
All	64.6	39.2	58.1	13.4	49.7	64.2	69.2	36.5
Matching	24.8	16.8	35.8	19.7	19.4	29.9	29.6	23.8
Neonatal	19.7	20.7	20.2	13.8	18.5	42.5	28.9	13.1
Preg.	14.4	11.5	16.0	20.8	20.7	25.7	34.6	25.6
Sociolog.	27.5	22.5	27.5	24.1	26.0	30.1	27.4	18.4
Growth-retarded babies								
All	32.9	32.9	27.8	25.4	32.5	41.3	32.8	28.4
Matching	25.0	18.4	23.9	21.7	16.9	21.2	15.7	20.5
Neonatal	16.2	13.7	16.7	12.8	26.7	42.6	34.8	24.5
Preg.	17.5	19.6	14.3	9.8	17.7	19.8	14.1	5.3
Sociolog.	28.3	30.4	27.1	19.6	23.7	32.4	21.1	29.6
Premature babies								
All	48.0	36.5	40.1	35.8	41.9	55.8	53.6	59.0
Matching	37.1	32.9	31.1	33.7	9.8	41.5	21.2	30.6
Neonatal	39.2	33.6	37.0	24.9	38.4	53.4	38.7	47.7
Preg.	33.4	33.4	30.4	12.8	38.6	40.5	34.6	51.9
Sociolog.	41.2	44.1	29.6	32.5	46.8	29.1	39.8	27.0

Table 9.14   Differentiating between LBW children who perform uniformly worse than their control ($n = 51$) and the remainder ($n = 79$). (a) Mean and standard deviations of IQ. (b) order of entry of variables

(a)

		Full	Verbal	Performance
Uniformly Worse Group	Mean	90.5	90.0	94.1
	SD	13.3	14.0	13.5
Remainder	Mean	106.1	105.6	106.3
	SD	22.4	22.3	22.2

(b)

Step	Variable	Wilks Lambda	Equiv. F	Sig.
1	Social class	0.954	5.386	0.022
2	Recreational activity	0.921	4.744	0.011
3	Interviewer's assessment	0.898	4.107	0.009
4	Smoking during pregnancy	0.872	3.963	0.005
5	Maternal delivery complic.	0.850	3.765	0.004
6	Gestational age	0.837	3.439	0.004

function. It can be seen that the three variables which provide most discriminative power between the two groups of children as defined are:

1. The social class of the LBW parents.
2. The recreational activity index of the parents.
3. The interviewer's assessment of the LBW mother.

Other (physiological) variables such as smoking patterns during pregnancy, maternal delivery complications, maternal age and parity are included in the discriminant function only after these social variables, because they provide less discriminative power.

Impairments in physical characteristics

The number of variables which appear with significant coefficients in sets of equations for physical development is even further reduced. No variable appears significantly in all sub-populations and indeed only three variables appear in more than one. These are:

1. The difference in maternal height, which appears positively in the equations for older mothers and for premature babies.
2. The difference in general nutritional status, which appears negatively in the equation for the whole population and for premature babies.
3. The difference in birthweight, which appears positively in the equations for young mothers and for both growth retarded and premature babies.

Correlations

Although the extent of the overlap is not the same as with the mental measurement, there is still considerable commonality between the sets of variables which have high simple correlation coefficients with the physical outcome characteristics. They will therefore be discussed as a triad (actual height, actual weight, actual head circumference) below:

1. Differences in birth weight between LBW and controls ($r = 0.34, 0.40, 0.41$), the lighter the LBW child relative to the control the larger the physical impairment.
2. Differences in maternal height ($r = 0.27, 0.14, 0.21$), the shorter the LBW mother relative to the control, the larger the physical impairment.
3. Attitudes to behaviour training of LBW parents ($r = 0.22, 0.024, 0.977$), the stricter the LBW parent, the smaller the impairment.
4. Differences in attitude to behaviour training ($r = 0.21, 0.019, 0.11$), the stricter the LBW parent relative to the control, the smaller the impairment.
5. Birth weight of the LBW child ($r = 0.20, 0.13, 0.14$), the lighter the LBW child, the larger the physical impairment.
6. Days spent in special care baby unit by LBW child ($r = -0.20, -3.2, -0.12$), the more days spent in the special care baby unit, the larger the physical impairment.

We note also the relatively large simple correlations of the child's actual weight positively with differences in maternal role preparation and the number of medical conditions specific to pregnancy, and negatively with differences in the neonatal problem index; and the child's actual head circumference positively with the number of uncompleted pregnancies experienced by the LBW mother and negatively with differences in the neonatal problem index and the previous obstetric history of the LBW mother.

Three of these correlations (those with differences in birth weight, differences in maternal height and birth weight of the LBW child) are simple to interpret: the smaller the baby or the mother, the smaller the child at age 10. The last correlation coefficient with the number of days spent in the special baby care unit reflects the severity of the child's medical condition at birth which may be a continuing disadvantage. The most unusual correlations are those between impairment and attitudes to behaviour training: *prima facie*, they suggest that a flexible attitude to behaviour training on the part of the parents is not universally a good thing. It will be interesting to see whether the same result appears in the multivariate analysis.

Regressions

The first point is that once again there is some complementary pairing of absolute values with difference scales. Thus, in the equations for head circumference, birth weight and differences in birth weight in the whole population, and gestational age and differences in gestational age appear in the equations for the whole population and for older mothers: while number of neonatal problems and differences in number of neonatal problems appear only in the equation for older mothers. In the equations for height, maternal height and differences in maternal height appear in the equation for older mothers and maternal age and differences in maternal age in the equation for premature babies.

There is also another type of pairing as between a variable and its difference scale when we look at the results *across* different populations. Thus in the equations for weight impairment, the absolute value of the variable 'medical conditions specific to pregnancy' enters the equation for older mothers and the difference scale for the whole population; and in the equations for height impairment, birth weight enters as an absolute value in the equation for premature babies and as a difference scale in the equations for the whole population. In what follows we have treated such effects as the same.

For the whole population, if we ignore the pairing of the absolute values and differences of birth weight and of gestational age, only one appears in at least two of the equations; thus the LBW sample are less physically impaired, the poorer their general nutritional status at birth compared to their controls. Otherwise, isolated variables appear in each of the three equations and, in particular, difference in parental attitudes to behaviour training only appears in one of the three equations.

When we divide the population into younger and older mothers, the difference in general nutritional status at birth remains in the equations for younger mothers but not for older mothers. Otherwise for younger mothers both difference in birth weight and difference in gestational age appear in all these equations *without* being paired with the absolute value variable—but their effects work in opposite directions. For older mothers, however, three variables appear consistently and with a positive impact on reducing impairment: that is, differences in maternal height, differences in birth weight and the number of maternal delivery complications. Whilst, therefore, the results for younger mothers are rather confusing, for older mothers there seem to be simple relationships between the birth event and subsequent physical development.

The split between growth retarded and premature babies is perhaps more convincing and the Chow test confirms this (Table 9.12). Once again, as with the equations for the absolute values, very few variables appear to influence the outcome amongst growth retarded babies and, in fact, the only variable to appear consistently is differences in birthweight, where LBW babies who are heavy relative to their controls are less impaired. However, considerably more variables appear consistently in at least two of the equations for premature babies: thus the LBW child is relatively less impaired, the taller the LBW mother is relative to her control, the less disparity in weight between the LBW child and control, the poorer the general nutritional status of the LBW child relative to the control, the more preparation for motherhood by the LBW mother relative to her control, and the more abortions the LBW mother has had relative to her control.

Discussion

The patterns are similar to those found with the absolute values of the variables.

If we examine the right hand side of Table 9.13 we can see that the neonatal variables are always the most important in the overall population and usually in each of the sub-populations. The exceptions are, however, interesting: thus, the pregnancy variables are the most important in the equations for weight and height amongst the older mothers and also in the premature babies, and the sociological variables are most important in the equation for weight amongst mothers of premature babies.

When we compare the patterns of significant variables between the sub-populations and the overall population, we can see more clearly that the problems in directly interpreting the results for the overall population can usually be resolved by splitting the population between growth retarded and premature babies. The division between younger and older mothers does not produce quite such convincing results and we suspect that this is because that is not the most relevant division when studying subsequent physical development, although there is clearly some overlap between a division according to age and a division according to growth retardation or pre-term delivery.

The pattern of significant coefficients suggests that the factors influencing subsequent physical development amongst growth retarded infants, on the whole, have not been captured by the kind of variables we have used in this analysis. On the other hand, the results for the premature group suggest that a well grown and nourished LBW baby will tend to be smaller at least up to age 10 years, although premature babies of taller mothers who have had previous pregnancies and have prepared for motherhood may catch up. It is also of interest to note that the general nutritional status of the infant at birth consistently influences subsequent head size and height but not weight.

Chapter 10

Main Findings and Implications for Practice and Research

R. ILLSLEY AND R.G. MITCHELL

INTRODUCTION

It is well known that physical status at birth (and especially birth weight) and the socio-economic environment into which a child is born (and especially the quality of parenting) are strongly associated with the child's subsequent intellectual and physical development. This knowledge is acted upon: thus substantial effort is put into the medical management of pregnancy so that a healthy baby is produced and many paramedical and social services are directed towards improving the infant's environment. It is also increasingly realized that the causal interrelationships between birth weight and its antecedents, the immediate postnatal environment, external influences during childhood, and intellectual and physical development are extremely complicated. It is for this reason that, despite considerable advances in gynaecological, obstetric, and paediatric knowledge and practices and a plethora of studies documenting the effects of a disadvantaged socio-economic environment upon infant development, argument and debate continue between those who would improve medical services and those who would emphasize the importance of social change.

The purpose of this study was to attempt to unravel at least some of this tangle by studying a total geographical population of LBW children, carefully matching them to a control population according to several variables, meticulously collecting information about both populations at the time of birth (1970), and reviewing them all at the age of 10 years.

In this chapter, we first report the main findings in terms of:

1. the differences at birth and at age 10 between LBW and control children; and

2. the relative influence of medical and sociological factors at birth upon intellectual and physical development at age 10.

Second, we draw out the main lessons both methodological and substantive from this research in terms of:

1. the utility and reliability of a case control study in this kind of investigation;
2. the different constellations of factors which influence the intellectual and physical development of LBW babies.

Finally, we discuss some of the implications for health care and social policy.

THE FINDINGS

Differences between LBW and control children

At birth

Rather tritely, the major difference between LBW infants and their controls is the difference in their birth weights. However, there are also physiological differences in their mothers: thus, when compared to the controls, the mothers of LBW infants showed these differences:

1. They were reproductively less efficient in the sense that they had more spontaneous abortions or induced terminations.
2. They had experienced more medical conditions specific to pregnancy, such as pre-eclamptic toxaemia and haemorrhage.
3. They had experienced more medical complications such as anaemia, gynaecological disorders, and respiratory or other infections.
4. They had also experienced more premature rupture of the membranes, more obstetric intervention, and longer labours (note that the proportions induced were the same).
5. They had more infants with low Apgar scores and infants with lower blood pressure than the controls.

On this basis, five indices were constructed in Chapter 5, viz.: the previous obstetric history index, medical conditions specific to pregnancy index, medical complications not specific to pregnancy index, maternal complications of delivery index, and neonatal problems index, each of which discriminates between the LBW and control groups.

At the same time, there appear to be considerable differences in the socio-cultural background of the LBW children as compared to their controls, even though they had been matched for social class. Thus, the analysis of the post-natal interview with the mother showed how, even on the basis of these relatively poor data, it proved possible to construct indices which differentiated between the LBW and the control children. It is, of course, difficult to draw conclusive inferences from, for example, the intentions about child-rearing expressed at the time of delivery as to what is actually done subsequently but, taken at face value, the indices reflect these differences:

1. The socio-cultural background of the LBW families was poorer than that of the control families.
2. The lifestyle in the LBW families was less varied in terms of entertainment and recreation than in the control families.
3. The LBW mothers had fewer aspirations and expectations than the control mothers.
4. The attitudes to behaviour training of LBW mothers were more rigid than those of the controls.
5. The LBW mother apportioned a slighter role to her husband in matters of child-rearing.
6. The LBW mother was less prepared for motherhood than the control mother.
7. The range of vocabulary, fluency of expression, and organization as assessed by the interviewer were poorer amongst the LBW mothers than amongst the controls.

It is, of course, unsurprising that the whole range of socio-cultural variation cannot be captured by a single indicator. The trouble is that, although this is often recognized in the literature, these other aspects are rarely quantified in detail.

At 10 years

We showed in Chapter 9 that, although there were differences between the LBW children and their controls, these were not very large. Thus, it was certainly true that children who had birth weights of 2500 g or less were, at age 10, lighter and shorter and had smaller heads when compared to their controls but the differences (1.9 kg, 3.3 cm and 0.7 cm, respectively) are small. The LBW children had more neurological disorders and other diseases than their controls. The onset of puberty also appeared to be slower among LBW children—especially those with birth weights less than 2000 g—when compared to their controls.

In respect of most aspects of physical development, children who weighed 2000 g or less at birth were at a disadvantage compared with heavier LBW children; the only important association between perinatal events and subsequent health status was that between neonatal hypoglycaemia and later mental handicap.

Our results show that LBW children performed less well on tests of intellectual development (performance and verbal IQ) at age 10 when compared to their controls and again the differences (5.0 and 3.1 points, respectively) are small. We should also remark that the LBW children had a greater incidence of educational subnormality than their controls.

The lighter LBW children (2000 g and below) tended to contribute most to the noted deficits; amongst the heavier LBW children, only the growth-retarded prematures exhibited intellectual impairment. Moreover, our non-manual children showed least intellectual impairment though this may be partly due to better matching with their controls in terms of socio-economic status.

Relation between medical and sociological factors at birth and outcome at age 10

A straightforward comparison of medical and sociological conditions at birth and physical and intellectual development at age 10 appeared to show that *impairment in intelligence* is related to very low birth weight regardless of other factors. Thus, amongst heavier LBW infants (2000 to 2500 g) growth-retardation has a significant influence in determining subsequent intelligence, the growth-retarded showing greater degrees of impairment. However, amongst the infants of very low birth weight (less than 2000 g), intellectual impairment appears to be a function of the low weight and unrelated to rate of growth or gestational age.

At the same time, it was found that a LBW child from a skilled manual family will, on average, have a higher intelligence than a control child from an unskilled family, suggesting that the effect of a disadvantaged environment outweighs that of low weight at birth.

Mothers of LBW children were generally less physically and mentally active and less well-informed than mothers in the control group. They were also either very young or very old relative both to controls and to the child-bearing population of women in general. Clearly the aetiology of low weight at birth is likely to be quite different in the two age groups, and the outcomes correspondingly different.

The preliminary findings mentioned briefly above suggest that the developmental processes are likely to differ between growth-retarded and premature children and, therefore, we have analysed those two groups separately where appropriate.

Regression analysis of the data on the LBW group shows that, for the young mother of an LBW infant, the child's later intelligence will be higher if the pregnancy is her first and there have been no previous abortions; if the nutritional status of the infant is good at birth; if the mother is flexible in her attitude to behaviour training; and if the social environment at the time of birth is good. In the case of the older mother, the child will be more intelligent if he is the first child and a boy and if his mother has made considerable preparation for motherhood; the fewer the days spent in intensive care and the older the mother, the higher the child's intelligence is likely to be.

The data on parity should be interpreted with care. Mothers having their first pregnancy over the age of 25 may be seen as a different social category from multiparae of the same age, who could include some who started their reproductive life at very young ages and who may now have several children. This also applies to the younger age group, where multiparae may include a proportion of young and rapid reproducers. Parity is thus a sociological as well as a physiological category.

When we consider the *physical characteristics* of the child, the relationships are not so clear-cut. The results confirm that both fetal growth retardation and early birth are associated with unsatisfactory subsequent growth but that the effects of birth before term are less on heavier babies born to older mothers who have not previously had an abortion. Otherwise there is little evidence of a consistent relationship between the various independent variables and later physical growth.

When the LBW group is compared with the control group, analysis of data shows that the intelligence of the LBW child is less impaired relative to that of his control if there was less difference in the number of neonatal problems between LBW and control; if the LBW mother was older than the control; if the LBW child was socio-culturally advantaged compared with the control; and if the LBW mother's attitude to behaviour training was less rigid than that of her counterpart.

The height of the LBW mother has a negative effect on IQ impairment amongst children who have suffered fetal growth retardation but not amongst children who were born early, suggesting that if a tall mother produces a growth-retarded infant, something is very far wrong.

THE LESSONS

The design of the study

The study population comprised only babies born in hospital but, since over 98 per cent of all births in Aberdeen took place in hospital during the period in question, this could reasonably be considered as a total geographically defined population study. The control child chosen was the next to be born who matched the LBW child in sex, maternal height, parity and smoking habits during pregnancy, and social class of husband. Of the 296 children in the combined index and control populations, 290 (98 per cent) were traced at age 10 years so that the follow-up was virtually complete.

Although we were thus able to 'find' controls at birth and trace both index and control children at age 10, there were a number of methodological difficulties endemic to this kind of study.

First, the case control design originated in the natural sciences and has been adopted by psychologists as providing one of the most powerful techniques for drawing conclusions about the effect of one or a small number of factors upon a variable of interest.

The technique was developed for the situation where an experimental treatment is applied to a target set of cases randomly chosen from within a larger population and the 'controls' are therefore simply another random subset of that same population.

The technique therefore provides the data analyst with the simple task of comparing the level or quantity of the experimental treatment with the differences in outcomes between the target and control case. The situation in our study is quite different; the LBW children were not randomly chosen from within a larger population: indeed they constituted the population of LBW children in Aberdeen that year so they do not naturally occur randomly within any larger population. The implication is that both the technical and the interpretive simplicity of the basic statistical method is lost. Thus, on the one hand, as we cannot assume that both the targets and controls are random sub-sets from a larger population, we have to allow for the possibility of covariation of factors which affect outcome *other than* the 'treatment' with the characteristic(s) which distinguish between the target and the control groups. Although this does not make statistical inference impossible it does make it much more complex. On the other hand, in a certain sense one can only unequivocally conclude that the 'treatment' *per se* 'makes a difference' if the causal process linking the initial and final values of the outcome variables is the same in both target and control groups. In a situation with covariation of the type described above, a purist might argue that as there are two different processes, then the question of the 'treatment' *per se* making a difference does not arise.

Both these problems were compounded by the impossibility of controlling for or even documenting the plethora of environmental influences operating between the neonatal period and the age of 10 years. Apart from the (relatively) straightforward possibility that such environmental influences may also covary in the way described above, there is also the possibility that a small initial difference may, via a process of social differentiation, be amplified within the same socio-cultural milieu.

There are several factors which one could cite as covarying both with the outcome and with membership of either the target or the control group. In this study, the two which were apparently the most important were:

1. The difference among LBW babies between those who were growth-retarded and those who were born early.
2. The difference between babies born to younger mothers (under 25 years) and older mothers (25 years +).

We shall be returning to the differences which have been observed between LBW and control children: suffice to say here that the factors do covary and that this is a weakness of the design which could, in principle, have been avoided, but it is difficult to foresee every possible covariant.

Second, the fact that a control group is not a naturally occurring sub-set of a larger population, means that one has to *search* for controls. The difficulty of this search depends, of course, upon the rigour of the criteria. In this case we were looking for the next baby born who weighed more than 2500 g and who matched the target LBW baby in terms of maternal height (to within 5 cm), the same parity, the same sex, whether or not the mother smoked during pregnancy, and the same social class of husband. Despite the relative tightness of our criteria, we were able to attain a near perfect match on all five criteria for 72 per cent of the target cases and a good match on four of the criteria for almost all the remainder (see Chapter 3 for a fuller discussion).

However, although we were able to fulfil the matching criteria we had chosen, the intention was to control for the possible *effect* of these five factors. The efficacy of this obviously depends on the sensitivity of the outcome measure to small variations in the matching criteria, or, of course, in factors which covary with these matching criteria. The analysis in Chapter 3 showed that there were definitional problems in deciding whether or not a mother had smoked during pregnancy and that the matching for maternal height was less than perfect but the main problem was with the matching for social class.

Again, the *intention* was to match the LBW infant with a control in terms of socio-economic background and, while we knew that the father's occupation is an inadequate surrogate for such varied attributes as cultural attitudes, material possessions and status in the community, we also know that 'social class' defined in this way has been and is widely used as a way of classifying people and families.

We used the Registrar General's classification of social class by paternal occupation because it is the most widely used yardstick of social status in Britain. However, we recognized that any tendency for the LBW group to rank lower than the controls within these broad occupational classes might confer some advantage on the controls in terms of the postnatal social environment. Comparison according to a number of social and socially-related criteria, grouped to form composite indices, revealed that the control group did indeed have a higher socio-economic status. It is also apparent that differences are by no means as simple as this statement implies and so data must be interpreted with caution: for example, the occupational classes have been shown to be extremely heterogenous and families in the RG's Classes IV and V may provide a more favourable child-rearing environment than apparently more privileged families.

Styles of reproduction, maturation, and growth

Since this study started, there has been a considerable volume of research on intra-uterine growth retardation, on neonatal pathology and on their joint implications for childhood development. As a result of this research, it has become accepted that babies who are growth-retarded are worse off in developmental terms than babies who, for whatever reasons, are born before term; and that VLBW infants (less than 2000 g) are worse off than other LBW infants (between 2000 and 2500 g).

It was not our purpose in undertaking this study to confirm yet again these results: we already knew—albeit with less evidence than today—that there were important differences between VLBW and other LBW children, and also between growth-retarded and pre-term children. The particular purpose of this study was to explore how these conditions interacted with other medical conditions and the social environment to affect intellectual and physical development at age 10.

If we look at the results for the LBW children both in isolation and in relation to their controls certain patterns emerge.

First, the results for intellectual development:

1. It is true that heavier LBW babies will do better than lighter, which confirms the importance of distinguishing VLBW from the other LBW infants (without, however, pointing to any particular dividing line). At the same time, relative to their controls, neither their birth weight nor the difference in birth weight from their controls affects the relative impairment of LBW children: rather, it is the presence or lack of neonatal problems and this is true whether the baby is growth-retarded or born before term.
2. Firstborn babies do better than others amongst LBW infants of older mothers, while the reverse is true amongst LBW babies born prematurely. Both results conform with knowledge about different kinds of reproductive careers, e.g. the *decision* of an older mother to start a family, and the relative preponderance of multiparae amongst mothers of prematurely born babies. At the same time if, relative to her control, the LBW mother has had more births, then the child is less impaired if she herself was young or if the baby was born prematurely.
3. Amongst the LBW group, the children of taller mothers do worse, especially if the child is growth-retarded, suggesting that when this happens something is really wrong. At the same time if, relative to her control, a mother is smaller then the child is less impaired.

All three of these findings are consistent with the contention that it is not the LBW in and of itself which makes the difference, in that *if the baby is otherwise healthy or if the LBW child is born to a mother who is more prone to pre-term delivery, then the impairment, both absolute and relative, is lower.*

Moreover, the conditions at birth contribute only part of the story. Even though we acknowledge that the postnatal questionnaire was unsatisfactory in several respects, we were able to distil from it a variety of indices to tap a range of socio-cultural and environmental factors, outlined below, which did appear consistently in both absolute and relative equations.

1. The more favourable the interviewer's assessment of the LBW mother, the better the outcome, both absolutely and relatively.
2. The better the socio-cultural environment of the LBW mother, the better the outcome amongst younger mothers; and the better her environment relative to the control, the less the impairment relative to the control in each of the sub-populations.
3. The more rigid the LBW mother's attitude to behaviour training, the better the outcome, while the nearer her attitude is to that of the control, the less the relative impairment.

The first two results are a clear demonstration that 'better' social conditions improve the likely outcome. The third result is making essentially the negative point that the mother who feels incompetent or unable to bring up her child is likely to create a worse developmental environment for the child. *Thus, in the child of low weight at birth, a positive social environment may offset the effect on subsequent intelligence of a number of initial disadvantages.*

The main finding about physical development is a negative one: that amongst growth-retarded babies, none or very few of the factors considered in this study, whether medical or social, have any influence at all on subsequent physical development. The most plausible interpretation of this negative result is that, whatever are the factors which determine the subsequent growth of growth-retarded children, they are relatively specific to the particular physiopathological causes of that same growth-retardation.

Among the other results for physical development, some are obvious enough. Thus:

1. Amongst older mothers and pre-term babies, the taller the LBW mother relative to her control, the larger is the LBW baby.
2. Amongst LBW babies, the heavier babies grow to be heavier and taller and this is also true relatively.

Some of the other results are at first surprising. Thus the fact that pre-term babies do better should probably be interpreted in terms of the relative normality of an LBW baby born early. This is reinforced by the fact that pre-term babies born to older mothers do better. At the same time, we note that the child does better if the mother has had no previous abortions and that obstetric intervention has an apparently beneficial effect.

In interpreting the findings we have to rely on our knowledge and judgement as to what should count as relatively normal birth given other conditions, but the combined results all point towards the same conclusion, viz. that *being of LBW is not a handicap if, for whatever combination of circumstances, the baby is an appropriate size given the mother's physique and the progress of the pregnancy.*

CONCLUSIONS RELEVANT TO HEALTH CARE

Now that so many other perinatal hazards have been eliminated in this country or their threat diminished, low birth weight with its implications for later outcome is the greatest single challenge to the obstetric and paediatric services. In recent years, improvements in the general health of the population and in medical practice have resulted in a change in the composition of the LBW population. More infants of very low birth weight are surviving and attention has consequently been focused on them because they are believed to be especially vulnerable. Nevertheless, all LBW infants are potentially at some risk and so in this study we have considered the whole LBW population, rather than concentrating exclusively on the important but numerically small sub-group of very low birth weight infants.

At the time of our survey, the perinatal mortality rate in Aberdeen was 18.9 per 1000 total births (1970), a figure lower than the national average for that year (Scotland 24.8, England and Wales 23.5). Thus we were dealing with an unusually healthy population of infants, largely free from the factors responsible for high perinatal mortality rates in other parts of the country, such as relatively poor standards of obstetric practice, inadequate neonatal care, and prevalence of infection. Since then there has been improvement in most areas of the United Kingdom, so that ten years later the perinatal mortality rates for Aberdeen, Scotland, and England and Wales were 13.5, 13.1, and 13.3, respectively (1980). The health status of the infants in our study was thus closely comparable with that of most infants in Britain today and we therefore believe that the conclusions to be drawn are currently valid for the whole country.

What are the implications of our findings for medical practice and research, especially in the fields of obstetrics and neonatology, and for social policies and research directed at expectant or new mothers?

The obstetrician will wish to claim our results as support for expanding clinical resources. It is true that we have confirmed that the lower average intelligence of children who weigh less than 2000 g at birth is related to that very low birth weight, so one could conclude that it must be a prime objective of management to prolong pregnancy in order to allow the fetus to grow to at least 2000 g. However, we have also shown that impairment relative to a normal birth weight child does not depend upon that low weight *per se* but upon the presence or absence of neonatal problems. Thus, our results would tend to suggest that, in cases where the fetus is growing slowly or adverse developments, such as differential slowing of growth of the fetal head (Creasy 1979), can be detected, then timely obstetric intervention may be beneficial.

Nevertheless, this rather begs the question: for it is clearly only a feasible clinical option if one can guarantee that the birth will take place in a well-staffed and equipped obstetric unit, where prompt action will be taken to avoid or minimize the effects of hypoxia or other known concomitants of brain damage, using continuous monitoring and other evaluation techniques: in this connection, the special vulnerability of the growth-retarded infant to complications of delivery should be remembered, as should the relationship between neonatal hypoglycaemia and subsequent neurological impairment. Such considerations clearly have large and potentially almost infinite resource implications.

On the other hand, it is apparent that investigation is needed into the aetiology of growth-retardation and the links between it and subsequent growth. Another area of research likely to prove fruitful is the elaboration of precisely what is meant by a baby being born the appropriate size for a given maternal conformation and progress during pregnancy. While adequate numbers of properly equipped obstetric units are essential, it would perhaps be more productive in the long term to allocate resources to this kind of research rather than to the over-lavish provision and equipment of hospital units.

At the same time we have emphasized that, if the LBW baby is born prematurely or to an older mother, his subsequent development may be perfectly normal. Clearly, therefore, although prophylactic measures are important, they should be adjusted to this possible normality. Indeed, one of the major findings of this study is that the disadvantages associated with being of low weight at birth are largely the result of an unfavourable social environment and can accordingly be reduced or prevented by improvements in that environment. Where the socio-cultural environment of the home is better, where the mother appears to be more competent and prepared for bringing up her children, then the outcome is better. In this respect our study repeats and confirms many previous suggestions and findings.

We conclude that, while better antenatal and postnatal care remain desirable, improvements in physical and intellectual outcomes for LBW children are substantially dependent upon improvements in the quality of the social environments into which the children are born and in which they grow and develop.

References

Ainsworth, M.D.S. (1962). 'The effects of maternal deprivation: a review of findings and controversy in the context of research strategy' in *Deprivation of Maternal Care: a Reassessment of its Effects*, Public Health Papers No. 14, World Health Organisation, Geneva.

Ainsworth, M.D.S., Bell, S.M., and Stayton, D.J. (1974). 'Infant – mother attachment and social development: socialization as a product of reciprocal responsiveness to signals' in *The Integration of a Child into a Social World* (Ed. M.P.M. Richards), Cox and Wyman, London.

Anastasi, A. (1961). *Psychological Testing*, 2nd edn, Macmillan, New York.

Apgar, V. (1953). 'A proposal for a new method of evaluation of the newborn infant', *Anaesthesia and Analgesia*, **32**, 260 – 267.

Ashworth, A.M., Neligan, G.A., and Rogers, J.E. (1959). 'Sphygmomanometer for the newborn', *Lancet*, **i**, 801 – 807.

Askham, J. (1975). *Fertility and Deprivation*, University Press, Cambridge.

Baird, D. (1962). 'Environmental and obstetrical factors in prematurity with special reference to experience in Aberdeen', *Bulletin of the World Health Organisation*, **26**, 291 – 295.

Baird, D. (1974). 'The epidemiology of low birth weight: changes in incidence in Aberdeen 1948 – 72', J. Biosoc. Sci., **6**, 323 – 341.

Barker D.J.P. (1966). 'Low intelligence and obstetric complications', *Brit. J. Prev. Soc. Med.*, **20**, 15–21.

Barker, D.J.P. and Edwards, J.H. (1967). 'Obstetric complications and school performance', *Brit. Med. J.*, **3**, 695 – 699.

Bartemeier, L. (1953). 'The contribution of the father to the mental health of the family', *Amer. J. Psychiat.*, **110**, 277 – 280.

Baruch, D.W. and Wilcox, J.A. (1944). 'A study of sex differences in preschool children's adjustment coexistent with interparental tensions', *J. Genet. Psychol.*, **61**, 281 – 303.

Bax, M. and Mac Keith, R. (1963). *Minimal Cerebral Dysfunction. Little Club Clinics in Developmental Medicine No. 10,* National Spastics Society/Heinemann, London.

Beintema, D.J. (1968). *A Neurological Study of Newborn Infants. Clinics in Developmental Medicine No. 28,* Heinemann, London.

Benson, L.G. (1968). *Fatherhood: a Sociological Perspective,* Random House, New York.

Biller, H.B. (1971). *Father, Child and Sex Role: Paternal Determinants of Personality Development,* Heath Lexington Books, Lexington, Massachusetts.

259

Biller, H.B. (1974). 'The father-infant relationship: some naturalistic observations', Unpublished Manuscript, University of Rhode Island.

Birch, H.G. and Gussow, J.D. (1970). *Disadvantaged Children: Health, Nutrition and School Failure,* Harcourt Brace and World, New York.

Black, D.A.K. (1980). *Inequalities in Health: Report of a Research Working Group,* Department of Health and Social Security, London.

Blanchard, R.W. and Biller, H.B. (1971). 'Father availability and academic performance among third grade boys', *Developmental Psychology,* **4**, 301 – 305.

Block, J., von der Lippe, A., and Block, J.H. (1973). 'Sex role and socialization patterns: some personality concomitants and environmental antecedents', *J. Consult. Clin. Psychol.,* **41**, 321 – 341.

Boldman, R. and Reed, D.M. (1977). 'Worldwide variations in low birth weight' in *The Epidemiology of Prematurity* (Ed. D.M. Reed and F.J. Stanley), Urban and Schwarzenberg, Baltimore, pp. 39 – 52.

Bowlby, J. (1952). *Maternal Care and Mental Health. WHO Monograph Series No. 2,* World Health Organisation, Geneva.

Bowlby, J. (1969). *Attachment and Loss, vol. I, Attachment,* Basic Books, New York.

Brazelton, T.B. (1973). *Neonatal Behavioural Assessment Scale. Clinics in Developmental Medicine No. 50,* Heinemann, London.

British Medical Journal (1979). 'Towards fewer handicapped children', *Brit. Med. J.,* **2**, 1458.

Brofenbrenner, U. (1975). 'Research on the effects of day care', Unpublished Manuscript, Cornell University.

Brown, C.P.T. (1977). 'Premature baby statistics', *Brit. Med. J.,* **1**, 1598.

Burt, C. (1955). 'The evidence for the concept of intelligence', *Brit. J. Educ. Psychol.,* **25**, 158 – 177.

Butcher, H.J. (1968). *Human Intelligence: its Nature and Assessment,* Methuen, London.

Butler, N.R. and Alberman, E.D. (1969). *British Perinatal Mortality Survey—Second Report: Perinatal Problems,* Livingstone, Edinburgh.

Butler, N.R. and Bonham, D.G. (1963). *British Perinatal Mortality Survey—First Report: Perinatal Mortality,* Livingstone, Edinburgh.

Carr-Hill, R. and Samphier, M. (1981). Personal communication.

Cater, J.I. (1978). *A Population Study of Low Birthweight Infants with Special Reference to Impaired Fetal Growth.* M.D. Thesis, University of Edinburgh.

Chamberlain, A. (1976). 'Planning versus fatalism', *J. Biosoc. Sci.,* **8**, 1 – 16.

Chamberlain, R., Chamberlain, G., Howlett, B., and Claireaux, A. (1975). *British Births 1970, volume I, The First Week of Life,* Heinemann, London.

Chaplin, N.W. (Ed.) (1977). *The Hospitals and Health Services Year Book 1977,* Institute of Health Service Administrators, London.

Chiswick, M.L., Davies, P., Bate, R., Dryburgh, E., and Gordon-Nesbitt, D. (1979). 'Regional organisation of neonatal intensive care in the North-West', *Brit. Med. J.,* **2**, 247 – 250.

Clarke-Stewart, K.A. (1973) 'Interactions between mothers and their young children: characteristics and consequences', *Mon. Soc. Res. Child Develop. No. 38* (Serial No. 153)

Clements, S.D. and Peters, J.E. (1962). 'Minimal brain dysfunctions in the school age child', *Arch. Gen. Psychiat.,* **6**, 185 – 197.

Cohen, J. (1959). 'The factorial structure of the WISC at ages 7 – 6, 10 – 6 and 13 – 6', *J. Consult. Psychol.,* **23**, 285 – 299.

Coleman, J.S. and U.S. National Center for Educational Statistics, (1966). *Equality of Educational Opportunity,* U.S. Government Printing Office, Washington D.C.

Cornblath, M., Joassin, G., Weisskopf, B., and Swiatek, K.R. (1966). 'Hypoglycemia in the newborn', *Pediat. Clin. N. Amer.,* **13**, 905 – 920.

Creasey, R.K. (1979). In *Obstetrical Decisions and Neonatal Outcome* (Ed. L. Gluck), Ross Laboratories, Columbus, Ohio.

Daily, W.J.R., Klaus, M., and Meyer, H.B.P. (1969). 'Apnea in premature infants: monitoring, incidence, heart rate changes and an effect of environmental temperature', *Pediatrics,* **43**, 510 – 518.

Dann, M., Levine, S.Z., and New, E.V. (1958). 'The development of prematurely born children with birth weights or minimal postnatal weights of 1000 g or less', *Pediatrics,* **22**, 1037 – 1053.

Davie, R., Butler, N.R., and Goldstein, H. (1972). *From Birth to Seven,* Longman, London.

Davies, D.P. (1978). 'The first feed of low birthweight infants', *Arch. Dis. Childh.,* **53**, 187 – 192.

Davies, D.P. and Evans, T.J. (1978). 'Nutrition and early growth of preterm infants', *Early Human Development,* **2**, 383 – 392.

Davies, D.P., Haxby, V., Herbert, S., and McNeish, A.S. (1979). 'When should preterm babies be sent home from neonatal units?, *Lancet,* **i**, 914 – 915.

Davies, P.A. (1980). 'Perinatal mortality', *Arch. Dis. Childh.,* **55**, 833 – 837.

Davies, P.A. and Stewart, A.L. (1975). 'Low birth weight infants: neurological sequelae and later intelligence', *Brit. Med. Bull.,* **31**, 85 – 91.

Davis, A. (1946). 'The motivation of the underprivileged worker' in *Industry and Society* (Ed. F. Whyte), McGraw Hill, New York.

Davis, A. and Havinghurst, R.J. (1946). 'Social class and color differences in child-rearing', *Amer. Sociol. Rev.,* **11**, 698 – 710.

Dawkins, M. and MacGregor, W.G. (1965). *Gestational Age, Size and Maturity. Clinics in Developmental Medicine No. 19,* Heinemann, London.

Dennis, J. (1978). 'Neonatal convulsions: aetiology, late neonatal status and long-term outcome', *Developmental Medicine and Child Neurology*, **20**, 143 – 158.

De Hirsch, K., Jansky, J., and Langford, W.S. (1966). 'Comparisons between prematurely and maturely born children at three age levels', *Amer. J. Orthopsychiat.,* **36**, 616 – 628.

De Souza, S.W. and Richards, B. (1978). 'Neurological sequelae in newborn babies after perinatal asphyxia', *Arch. Dis. Childh.,* **53**, 564 – 569.

Dinwiddie, R., Mellor, D.H., Donaldson, S.H.C., Tunstall, M.E. and Russell, G. (1974). 'Quality of survival after artificial ventilation of the newborn', *Arch. Dis. Childh.,* **49**, 703 – 710.

Donnelly, J.F., Flowers, C.E., Creadick, R.N., Wells, H.B., Greenberg, B.G., and Surles, K.B. (1964). 'Maternal, fetal and environmental factors in prematurity', *Amer. J. Obstet. Gynec.,* **88**, 918 – 931.

Douglas, J.W.B. (1956). 'Mental ability and school achievement of premature children at 8 years of age', *Brit. Med. J.,* **1**, 1210 – 1214.

Douglas, J.W.B. (1960). 'Premature children at primary schools', *Brit. Med. J.,* **1**, 1008 – 1013.

Douglas, J.W.B. and Blomfield, J.M. (1958). *Children under Five,* Allen and Unwin, London.

Douglas, J.W.B. and Gear, R. (1976). 'Children of low birthweight in the 1946 national cohort', *Arch. Dis. Childh.,* **51**, 820 – 827.

Drage, J.S. and Berendes, H. (1966). 'Apgar scores and outcome of the newborn', *Pediat. Clin. N. Amer.,* **13**, 635 – 643.

Drage, J.S., Kennedy, C., Berendes, H., Schwarz, B.K., and Weiss, W. (1966). 'The Apgar score as an index of infant morbidity—a report from the Collaborative Study of Cerebral, Palsy', *Developmental Medicine and Child Neurology*, **8**, 141 – 148.

Drillien, C.M. (1964). *The Growth and Development of the Prematurely Born Infant*, Livingstone, Edinburgh.

Drillien, C.M. and Drummond, M.B. (1977). *Neurodevelopmental Problems in Early Childhood*, Blackwell, Oxford.

Drillien, C.M., Thomson, A.J.M. and Burgoyne, K. (1980). 'Low birthweight children at early school age: a longitudinal study', *Development Medicine and Child Neurology*, **22**, 26–47.

Dubowitz, L.M.S., Dubowitz, V., and Goldberg, C. (1970). 'Clinical assessment of gestational age in the newborn infant', *J. Pediat.*, **77**, 1–10.

Dunn, P. and Speidel, B.D. (1980). 'Comparison of neonatal management methods for very low birthweight babies', *Brit. Med. J.*, **281**, 1489–1490.

Eaves, L.C., Nuttall, J.C., Klonoff, H., and Dunn, H.G. (1970). 'Developmental and psychological test scores in children of low birthweight', *Pediatrics*, **45**, 9–20.

Farr, V., Kerridge, D.F., and Mitchell, R.G. (1966a). 'The value of some external characteristics in the assessment of gestational age at birth', *Developmental Medicine and Child Neurology*, **8**, 657–660.

Farr, V., Mitchell, R.G., Neligan, G.A., and Parkin, J.M. (1966b). 'The definition of some external characteristics used in the assessment of gestational age in the newborn infant', *Developmental Medicine and Child Neurology*, **8**, 507–511.

Field, J.G. (1960). 'Two types of tables for use with Wechsler's Intelligence scales', *J. Clin. Psychol.*, **16**, 3–7.

Finnstrom, O. (1971). 'Studies on maturity in newborn infants. III. Neurological examination', *Neuropediatrie*, **3**, 72–96.

Finnstrom, O. (1972). 'Studies on maturity in newborn infants', *Acta paediatrica Scandinavica*, **61**, 33–41.

Fitzhardinge, P.M. and Ramsay, M. (1973). 'The improving outlook for the small prematurely born infant', *Developmental Medicine and Child Neurology*, **15**, 447–459.

Fitzhardinge, P.M. and Steven, E.M. (1972). 'The small-for-date infant. II. Neurological and intellectual sequelae', *Pediatrics*, **50**, 50–57.

Francis-Williams, J. and Davies, P.A. (1974). 'Very low birthweight and later intelligence', *Developmental Medicine and Child Neurology*, **16**, 709–728.

Franco, S. and Andrews, B.F. (1977). 'Reduction of cerebral palsy by neonatal intensive care', *Pediat. Clin. N. Amer.*, **24**, 639–649.

Freeberg, N.E. and Payne, D.T. (1967). 'Dimensions of parental practice concerned with cognitive development in the preschool child', *J. Genetic Psychol.*, **111**, 245–261.

Freud, S. (1940). *An Outline of Psychoanalysis*, Norton, New York.

General Register Office, London (1960). *Classification of Occupations*, HMSO, London.

General Register Office, Edinburgh (1971). *Census (Scotland): County Report for Aberdeen City*, HMSO, Edinburgh.

Goldstein, H. and Peckham, C. (1976). 'Birthweight, gestation, neonatal mortality and child development' in *The Biology of Fetal Growth*, (Eds D.F. Roberts and A.M. Thomson), Symposium of the Society for the Study of Human Biology, No. 15, pp. 81–108.

Goldstein, K.M., Caputo, D.V., and Taub, H.B. (1976). 'The effects of prenatal and perinatal complications on development at one year of age', *Child Development*, **47**, 613–621.

Grampian Regional Council: Department of Physical Planning (1980). *Grampian Population Forecasts*, Grampian Regional Council, Aberdeen.

Gregory, G.A., Kitterman, J.A., Phibbs, R.H., Tooley, W.H., and Hamilton, W.K. (1971). 'Treatment of the idiopathic respiratory distress syndrome with continuous positive airway pressure', *New Eng. J. Med.*, **284**, 1333–1340.

Hall, R.T. and Oliver, T.K. (1971). 'Aortic blood pressure in infants admitted to a neonatal intensive care unit', *Amer. J. Dis. Children*, **121**, 145–147.

Hanushek, E.A. and Jackson, J.E. (1977). *Statistical Methods for Social Scientists*, Academic Press, New York, pp. 124–129.

Harper, P.A., Fischer, L.K., and Rider, R.V. (1959). 'Neurological and intellectual status of prematures at three to five years of age', *J. Pediat.*, **55**, 679–690.

Harper, P.A. AND Wiener, G. (1965). 'Sequelae of low birthweight', *Ann. Rev. Med.*, **16**, 405–420.

Hess, R.D. and Torney, J.V. (1967). *The Development of Political Attitudes to Children*, Aldine, Chicago.

Hirata, T., Epcar, J.T., Walsh, A., Mednick, J., Harris, M., McGinnis, M.S., Sehring, S., and Papedo, G. (1983). 'Survival and outcome of infants 501 to 750 gm: a six-year experience', *J. Pediatr.*, **102**, 741–748.

Hoffman, W.S. (1937). 'A rapid photo-electric method for the determination of glucose in blood and urine', *J. Biol. Chem.*, **120**, 51–56.

Horwood, S.P., Boyle, M.H., Torrance, G.W. and Sinclair, J.C. (1982). 'Mortality and morbidity of 500- to 1,499-gram birthweight infants live born to residents of a defined geographic region before and after neonatal intensive care', *Pediatrics*, **69**, 613–620.

Houlsby, W.T. and Lloyd, D.J. (1980). 'Comparison of neonatal management methods for very low birthweight babies', *Brit. Med. J.*, **281**, 1489.

Hughes-Davies, T.H. (1981). 'Comparison of neonatal management methods for very low birthweight babies', *Brit. Med. J.*, **282**, 224.

Illsley, R. (1966). 'Early prediction of perinatal risk', *Proc. Roy. Soc. Med.*, **59** 181–184.

Illsley, R. (1967). 'Family growth and its effects on the relationship between obstetric factors and child functioning' in *Social and Genetic Influences on Life and Death* (Eds Lord Platt and A.S. Parkes), Oliver and Boyd, Edinburgh.

Illsley, R. (1980). *Professional and Public Health: Sociology in Health and Medicine*, Nuffield Provincial Hospitals Trust, London.

Illsley, R., Finlayson, A., and Thompson, B. (1963). 'The motivation and characteristics of internal migrants', *Millbank Memorial Fund Quarterly*, **41**, 115–144 and 217–248.

Isaacs, S. (1932). *The Nursery Years*, Routledge and Kegan Paul, London.

Jones, R.A.K., Cummins, M., and Davies, P.A. (1979) 'Infants of very low birthweight: a 15 year analysis', *Lancet*, **i**, 1332–1335.

Jordan, B.E., Radin, N., and Epstein, A. (1975). 'Paternal behavior and intellectual functioning in preschool boys and girls', *Develop. Psychol.*, **11**, 407–408.

Kagan, J. and Tulkin, S. (1971). 'Social class differences in childrearing during the first year' in *The Origins of Human Social Relations* (Ed. H.R. Schaffer), Academic Press, New York.

Kiely, J.L. and Paneth, N. (1981). 'Follow-up studies of low birthweight infants', *Developmental Medicine and Child Neurology*, **23**, 96–100.

Kitchen, W.H., Rickards, A., Ryan, M.M., McDougall, A.B., Billson, F.A., Keir, E.H., and Naylor, F.D. (1979). 'A longitudinal study of very low-birthweight infants. II. Results of controlled trial of intensive care and incidence of handicaps', *Developmental Medicine and Child Neurology*, **21**, 582–589.

Klein, J. (1965). *Samples from English Cultures*, Vol. II, Routledge and Kegan Paul, London.

Knobloch, H., Rider, R., Harper, P., and Pasamanick, B. (1956). 'Neuropsychiatric sequelae of prematurity', *J. Amer. Med. Ass.*, **161**, 581–585.

Koenigsberger, M.R. (1966). 'Judgment of fetal age. I. Neurologic evaluation', *Pediat. Clin. N. Amer.*, **13**, 823–833.

Kohn, M.L. and Carroll, E.E. (1960). 'Social class and the allocation of parental responsibilities', *Sociometry*, **23**, 372–392.

Koppitz, E.M. (1964). *The Bender Gestalt Test for Young Children*, Grune and Stratton, New York.

Kreisberg, L. (1963). 'The relationship between socio-economic rank and behaviour', *Social Problems*, **10**, 334–353.

Lamb, M.E. (1975). 'Infant attachment to mothers and fathers', *Proc. Soc. Res. Child Develop., Denver 1975*, Unpublished Manuscript.

Lamb, M.E. (1976). 'Parent-infant interaction in eight month olds', *Child Psychiat. and Hum. Develop.*, **7**, 56–63.

Lancet Editorial (1980). 'The fate of the baby under 1501 g. at birth', *Lancet*, **i**, 461–463.

Latis, G.O., Simionato, L., and Ferraris, G. (1981). 'Clinical assessment of gestational age in the newborn infant: comparison of two methods', *Early Human Development*, **5**, 29–37.

Levene, M.I. and Dubowitz, M.S. (1982). 'Low birth weight babies, long-term follow-up', *Brit. J. Hospt. Med.*, **28**, 487–493.

Lewis, O. (1966). 'The culture of poverty', *Scientific American*, **251**, 4:19–25.

Littell, W.M. (1960). 'The Wechsler Intelligence Scale for Children', *Psychol. Bull.*, **57**, 132–156.

Littman, B. and Parmelee, A.H. (1978). 'Medical correlates of infant development., *Pediatrics*, **61**, 470–474.

Lubchenco, L.O., Hansman, C., Dressler, M., and Boyd, E. (1963). 'Intra-uterine growth as estimated from liveborn birthweight data at 24 to 42 weeks of gestation', *Pediatrics*, **32**, 793–800.

Lubchenco, L.O., Horner, F.A., Reed, L.H., Hix, I.E., Metcalf, D., Cohig, R., Elliott, H.C., and Bourg, M. (1963). 'Sequelae of premature birth', *Amer. J. Dis. Children*, **106**, 101–115.

Lubchenco, L.O., Papadopoulos, M.D., and Searls, D. (1972). 'Long-term follow-up studies of prematurely born infants. II. Influence of birthweight and gestational age on sequelae', *J. Pediat.*, **80**, 509–512.

Lynn, D.B. (1974). *The Father: His Role in Child Development*, Brooks/Cole, Monterey, California.

McClelland, D.C., Atkinson, J.W., and Lowell, E.L. (1953). *The Achievement Motive*, Appleton Century Crofts, New York.

McDonald, A.D. (1964). 'Intelligence in children of very low birth weight', *Brit. J. Prev. Soc. Med.*, **18**, 59–74.

McGraw, M.B. (1943). *The Neuromuscular Maturation of the Human Infant*, Hafner, New York.

McKeown, T. (1970). 'Prenatal and early postnatal influences on measured intelligence', *Brit. Med. J.*, **3**, 63–67.

Marriage, K.J. and Davies, P.A. (1977). 'Neurological sequelae in children surviving mechanical ventilation in the neonatal period', *Arch. Dis. Childh.*, **52**, 176–182.

Mitchell, R.G. and Farr, V. (1965). 'The meaning of maturity and the assessment of maturity at birth' in *Gestational Age, Size and Maturity. Clinics in Developmental Medicine No. 19*, Heinemann, London.

Morley, G., Dawson, A., and Marks, V. (1968). 'Manual and autoanalyser methods for measuring blood glucose using guaiacum and glucose oxidase', *Proc. Ass. Clin. Biochem.*, **5**, 42–47.

Morris, J.N. and Heady, J.A. (1955). 'Social and biological factors in infant mortality. V. Mortality in relation to the father's occupation', *Lancet*, **i**, 554–560.

Neligan, G.A., Kolvin, I., Scott, D.M., and Garside, R.F. (1976). *Born too Soon or Born too Small. Clinics in Developmental Medicine No. 61*, Heinemann, London.

Nelson, K.B. and Ellenberg, J.H. (1979). 'Neonatal signs as predictors of cerebral palsy', *Pediatrics*, **64**, 225–232.

Newland, T.E. and Smith, P.A. (1967). 'Statistically significant differences between sub-test scaled scores on the WISC and the WAIS', *J. School Psychol.*, **5**, 122–127.

Newson, J. and Newson, E. (1963). *Patterns of Infant Care in an Urban Community*, Allen and Unwin, London.

Newson, J. and Newson, E. (1968). *Four Years Old in an Urban Community*, Allen and Unwin, London.

Njiokiktjien, C. and Kurver, P. (1980). 'Predictive value of neonatal neurological examination for cerebral function in infancy', *Developmental Medicine and Child Neurology*, **22**, 736–747.

O'Hagan, J.E., Hamilton, T., Le Breton, E.G., and Shaw, A.E. (1957). 'Human serum bilirubin: an immediate method of determination and its application to the establishment of normal values', *Clin. Chem.*, **3**, 609–623.

Paine, R.S. and Oppé, T.E. (1966). *Neurological Examination of Children. Clinics in Developmental Medicine Nos. 20/21*, Heinemann, London.

Paine, R.S., Werry, J.S., and Quay, H.C. (1968). 'A study of minimal cerebral dysfunction', *Developmental Medicine and Child Neurology*, **10**, 505–520.

Paneth, N., Kiely, J.L., Stein, Z., and Susser, M. (1981). 'Cerebral palsy and newborn care. III. Estimated prevalence rates of cerebral palsy under differing rates of mortality and impairment of low-birthweight infants', *Developmental Medicine and Child Neurology*, **23**, 801–817.

Pape, K.E., Buncic, R.J., Ashby, S., and Fitzhardinge, P.M. (1978). 'The status at two years of low birthweight infants born in 1974 with birth weights of less than 1,001 gm.', *J. Pediat.*, **92**, 253–260.

Parkin, J.M., Hey, E.N., and Clowes, J.S. (1976). 'Rapid assessment of gestational age at birth', *Arch. Dis. Childh.*, **51**, 259–263.

Parsons, T. (1958). 'Social structure and the development of personality: Freud's contribution to the integration of psychology and sociology', *Psychiatry*, **21**, 321–340.

Pasamanick, B., Knobloch, H., and Lilienfeld, A.M. (1956). 'Socioeconomic status and some precursors of neuropsychiatric disorder', *Amer. J. Orthopsychiat.*, **26**, 594–601.

Pedersen, F.A., Rubenstein, J., and Yarrow, L.J. (1973). 'Father absence in infancy', *Proc. Soc. Res. Child Develop., Philadelphia 1973*, Unpublished Manuscript.

Prechtl, H.F.R. (1977). *The Neurological Examination of the Full-Term Newborn Infant*, 2nd edn. *Clinics in Developmental Medicine No. 63*, Heinemann, London.

Radin, N. (1972). 'Father-child interaction and the intellectual functioning of four-year-old boys', *Develop. Psychol.*, **6**, 353–361.

Rawlings, G., Reynolds, E.O.R., Stewart, A., and Strang, L.B. (1971). Changing prognosis for infants of very low birth weight', *Lancet*, **i**, 516–519.

Record, R.G., McKeown, T., and Edwards, J.H. (1969). 'The relation of measured intelligence to birth weight and duration of gestation', *Ann. Hum. Genet., Lond.*, **33**, 71–79.

Reynolds, G.J. (1980). 'Comparison of neonatal management methods for very low birthweight babies', *Brit. Med. J.*, **281**, 1640.

Reynolds, O. and Stewart, A. (1980). 'Comparison of neonatal management methods for very low birthweight babies', *Brit. Med. J.*, **281**, 1488–1489.

Robinson, N.M. and Robinson, H.B. (1965). 'A follow-up study of children of low birth weight and control children at school age', *Pediatrics*, **35**, 425–433.

Robinson, R.J. (1966). 'Assessment of gestational age by neurological examination', *Arch. Dis. Childh.*, **41**, 437–447.

Rona, R.J., Swan, A.V., and Altman, D.G. (1978). 'Social factors and height of primary schoolchildren in England and Scotland', *J. Epidem. Comm. Health*, **32**, 147–154.

Rubin, R.A., Rosenblatt, C., and Balow, B. (1973). 'Psychological and educational sequelae of prematurity', *Pediatrics*, **52**, 352–363.

Rutter, M. (1971). 'Parent-child separation: psychological effects on the children', *J. Child Psychol. Psychiat.*, **12**, 233–260.

Rutter, M. (1972). *Maternal Deprivation Reassessed*, Penguin, Harmondsworth.

Rutter, M. (1979). 'Maternal deprivation 1972–78: new findings, new concepts, new approaches', *Child Develop.*, **50**, 283–305.

Saint-Anne Dargassies, S. (1974). *Le Développement Neurologique du Nouveau-né à Terme et Prématuré*, Masson, Paris.

Sameroff, A.J. and Chandler, M.J. (1975). 'Reproductive risk and the continuum of caretaking casualty', in *Review of Child Development 4* (Eds F.D. Horowitz, M. Hetherington, S. Scarr-Salapatek, and G. Siegal), University Press, Chicago.

Samphier, M.L. and Thompson, B. (1981). 'The Aberdeen maternity and neonatal data bank' in *Prospective Longitudinal Research* (Eds S.A. Mednick and A.E. Baert), University Press, Oxford.

Sattler, J.M. (1974). *Assessment of Children's Intelligence*, Saunders, Philadelphia.

Schaffer, H.R. and Emerson, P.E. (1964). 'The development of social attachments in infancy', *Mon. Soc. Res. Child Develop. No. 29* (Serial No. 94).

Schain, R.J. (1973). *Neurology of Childhood Learning Disorders*, Williams and Wilkins, Baltimore.

Scheiner, A.P. (1980). 'Perinatal asphyxia: factors which predict developmental outcome', *Developmental Medicine and Child Neurology*, **22**, 102–104.

Scott, H. (1976). 'Outcome of very severe birth asphyxia', *Arch. Dis. Childh.*, **51**, 712–716.

Scottish Home and Health Department (1979). *Scottish Health Statistics 1978*, SHHD, Edinburgh.

Sears, R.R., Maccoby, E.E., and Levin, H. (1957). *Patterns of Child Rearing*, Row Peterson, Evanston.

Sheridan, M.D. (1976a). *Manual for the Stycar Vision Tests*, 3rd edn, National Foundation for Educational Research, London.

Sheridan, M.D. (1976b). *Manual for the Stycar Hearing Tests*, 3rd edn, National Foundation for Educational Research, London.

Silverman, W.A. (1961). *Dunham's Premature Infants*, 3rd edn, Hoeber, New York.

Simmons, M.A., Adcock, E.W., Bard, H., and Battaglia, F.C. (1974). 'Hypernatremia and intracranial hemorrhage in neonates', *New Engl. J. Med.*, **291**, 6–10.

Spinley, B.M. (1953). *The Deprived and the Privileged*, Greenwood Press, London.

Spock, B. (1957). *Baby and Child Care*, Duell Sloane and Pearce, New York.

Stanley, F.J. and Alberman, E.D. (1978). 'Infants of very low birth weight. I. Perinatal factors affecting survival', *Developmental Medicine and Child Neurology*, **20**, 300–312.

Steiner, E.S., Sanders, E.M., Phillips, E.C.K., and Maddock, C.R. (1980). 'Very low birthweight children at school age: a comparison of neonatal management methods', *Brit. Med. J.*, **281**, 1237–1240.

Stewart, A. and Turcan, D. (1977). 'Continuing improvement in the prognosis for infants who weighed ≤ 1500 gm at birth', *Pediatric Research*, **11**, 1025.

Stewart, A.L. and Reynolds, E.O.R. (1974). 'Improved diagnosis for infants of very low birth weight', *Pediatrics*, **54**, 724–735.

Stewart, A.L., Reynolds, E.O.R., and Lipscomb, A.P. (1981). 'Outcome for infants of very low birth weight: survey of world literature', *Lancet*, **i**, 1038–1041.

Tanner, J.M. (1962). *Growth at Adolescence*, Blackwell, Oxford.

Teele, J.E., Blake, P., Sawzin, M., and Abeles, G. (1978). 'Sample maintenance and ethical issues in a longitudinal research study', *Proc. Amer. Sociol. Ass., San Francisco 1978*, Unpublished Manuscript.

Thompson, B. (1977). 'Problems of abortion in Britain: Aberdeen, a case study', *Population Studies*, **31**, 143–154.

Thompson, T. and Reynolds, J. (1977). 'The results of intensive care therapy for neonates', *J. Perinatal Med.*, **5**, 59–75.

Thomson, A.J., Searle, M., and Russell, G. (1977). 'Quality of survival after severe birth asphyxia, *Arch. Dis. Child.*, **52**, 620–626.

Thomson, A.M. and Billewicz, W.Z. (1963). 'Nutritional status, maternal physique and reproductive efficiency', *Proc. Nutr. Soc.*, **22**, 55–60.

Thomson, A.M., Billewicz, W.Z., and Hytten, F.E. (1968). 'The assessment of fetal growth', *J. Obstet. Gynaec. Brit. Cwlth*, **75**, 903–916.

Touwen, B.C.L. and Prechtl, H.F.R. (1970). *The Neurological Examination of the Child with Minor Nervous Dysfunction. Clinics in Developmental Medicine No. 38*, Heinemann, London.

Touwen, B.C.L. and Sporrel, T. (1979). 'Soft signs and MBD', *Developmental Medicine and Child Neurology*, **21**, 528–530.

Truby King, F. (1937). *Feeding and Care of the Baby*, Oxford University Press, London.

Tunstall, M.E., Cater, J.I., Thomson, J.S., and Mitchell, R.G. (1968). 'Ventilating the lungs of newborn infants for prolonged periods', *Arch. Dis. Childh.*, **43**, 486–497.

Turcan, D., Rawlings, G., and Stewart, A. (1977). 'School performance at 8 years of infants who weighed ≤ 1500 g. at birth', *Pediatric Research*, **11**, 1025.

Usher, R. (1963). 'Reduction of mortality from respiratory distress syndrome of prematurity with early administration of intravenous glucose and sodium bicarbonate', *Pediatrics*, **32**, 966–975.

Usher, R., McLean, F., and Scott, K.E. (1966). 'Judgment of fetal age. II. Clinical significance of gestational age and an objective method for its assessment'. *Pediat. Clin. N. Amer.*, **13**, 835–848.

Vohr, B.R. and Hack, M. (1982). 'Developmental follow-up of low-birth-weight infants', *Pediat. Clin. N. Amer.*, **29**, 1441–1454.

Volpe, J.J. (1979). 'Value of the neonatal neurologic examination', *Pediatrics*, **64**, 547–548.

Werner, E., Simonian, K., Bierman, J.M., and French, F.E. (1967). 'Cumulative effect of perinatal complications and deprived environment on physical, intellectual and social development of pre-school children', *Pediatrics*, **39**, 490–505.

Wesley, J. (1872). *Works*, Wesleyan Conference Office, London.

Westgren, M., Ingemarsson, I., Ahlström, H., Lindroth, M., and Svenningsen, N.W. (1982). 'Delivery and long-term outcome of very low birth weight infants'. *Acta Obst. Gynecol. Scand.*, **61**, 25–30.

Wiener, G. (1968). 'Scholastic achievement at age 12–13 years of prematurely born infants', *J. Spec. Educat.*, **2**, 237–250.

Wiener, G. (1970). 'The relationship of birthweight and length of gestation to intellectual development at ages 8 to 10 years', *J. Pediat.*, **76**, 694–699.

Wiener, G., Rider, R.V., Oppel, W.C., Fischer, L.K., and Harper, P.A. (1965). 'Correlates of low birth weights: psychological status at six to seven years of age', *Pediatrics*, **35**, 434–444.

Wiener, G., Rider, R.V., Oppel, W.C., and Harper, P.A. (1968). 'Correlates of low birth weight: psychological status at eight to ten years of age', *Pediatric Research*, **2**, 110–118.

Willmott, P. and Young, M. (1960). *Family and Class in a London Suburb*, Routledge and Kegan Paul, London.

World Health Organisation (1978). *Report on Social and Biological Effects on Perinatal Mortality*, WHO Statistical Publishing House, Budapest.

Wright, F.H., Blough, R.R., Chamberlain, A., Ernest, T., Halstead, W.C., Meier, P., Moore, R.Y., Naunton, R.F. and Newell, F.W. (1972). 'A controlled follow-up study of small prematures born from 1952 through 1956', *Amer. J. Dis. Children*, **124**, 506–521.

Zeller, R.A. and Carmines, E.G. (1978). *Statistical Analysis of Social Data*, Rand-McNally Co., Chicago.

Index

269